PLANT BASED DIET
COOKBOOK
FOR SENIORS

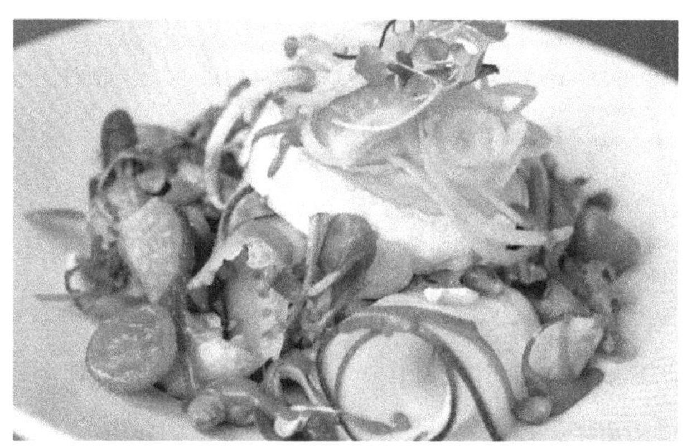

The Complete Simple & Delicious Vegan Recipes with Gluten-Free and Nutritious Meals for Healthy Living

Maria J. Kirby

Dear Seniors,

First and foremost, I want to extend my heartfelt gratitude to you for choosing this cookbook. In a shelf filled with countless options, I am deeply honored that you have entrusted me to be your guide on your plant-based journey.

Within the pages of this cookbook, you'll find a treasure trove of simple & delicious recipes, practical tips, and valuable insights crafted specifically for you for choosing this path to a healthier and more vibrant life through plant-based eating.

As you read further, I encourage you to embrace the joy of cooking, the nourishment of wholesome ingredients, and the empowerment of taking charge of your health and well-being. May this cookbook serve as a source of inspiration, comfort, and culinary delight as you go through this enriching journey towards a happier, healthier you. With deepest gratitude and warmest wishes.

KINDLY SCAN THIS CODE TO GET MORE HEALTHY COOKBOOKS FROM THIS AUTHOR

TABLE OF CONTENTS

Healthy Dessert Options for Occasional Indulgence

Snack Ideas for Boosting Energy and Satiety

Sweet and Savory Treats for Special Occasions

Hydrating Beverage Options

Importance of Social Connection and Community

14 DAYS MEAL PLAN

Shopping list Ingredients

Conclusion

Bonus 1: Nutritional Information For Meals

EXCLUSIVE BONUSES

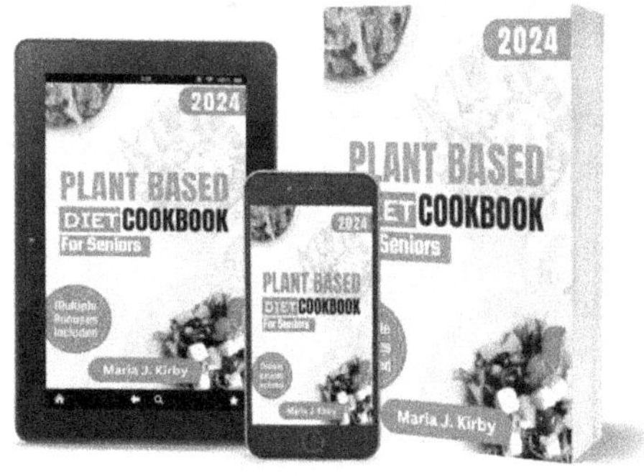

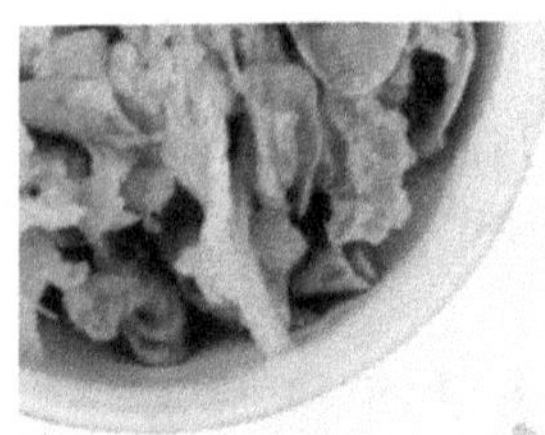

2024

PLANT BASED

DIET COOKBOOK

For Seniors

Multiple Bonuses Included

Maria J. Kirby

INTRODUCTION

I observed my dear Grandma Jane's health failing in spite of the prescription drugs and diet that her physician had prescribed, as she battled recurrent heart attacks. I knew there had to be a better way, so it hurt to watch her suffer. Based on my extensive background as a nutritionist, I recognized the fundamental problem: she required a significant change in her diet.

That is when I made the decision to act independently. I worked hard and with love to create "The Plant-Based Diet Cookbook especially for Seniors," a unique gift for her. It was a labor of love, chock full of advice and recipes to help her feel better and be more energetic.

I sat by her side and talked about the advantages of switching to a plant-based diet. I explained how my own family had benefited greatly from plant-based and vegan diets, and how she might experience a dramatic improvement in her health as a result of this shift. A week later, Grandma Jane came up to me, her eyes full of happy tears. She told me about her accomplishment and expressed her sincere thanks for the gift I had given her. The book's recipes had become her go-to guide for nutrient-rich living that supported her heart health, helped her control her weight, strengthened her bones, and improved her digestion.

Grandma Jane became stronger and more energetic every day, which is evidence of the benefits of a plant-based diet. She excitedly shared the recipes with her senior friends, introducing them to the many benefits of a plant-based diet. I experienced a deep sense of satisfaction knowing that I had improved her life as I saw her flourish. There was no turning back now that we had set out on this path of healing and transformation together. With love and gratitude, we embraced the gift of health and vitality that the plant-based diet had bestowed upon us.

The phrase "plant-based diet" has become increasingly well-known in recent years, drawing interest from people all over the world who are concerned about their health. However, its significance goes far beyond style, providing a significant paradigm shift regarding nutrition and wellness. The fundamental idea behind a plant-based diet is to honor the abundant abundance of nature by consuming whole, unprocessed plant-based foods such as fruits, vegetables, grains, legumes, nuts, and seeds. It's a lifestyle based on kindness toward our bodies and the environment, not just a food decision.

Scientific research supports the plant-based diet's potential to support longevity and optimal health. Several studies have demonstrated these benefits. People can nourish their bodies from the inside out, building resilience against chronic diseases and improving general vitality, by adopting a plant-based diet high in fiber, antioxidants, and essential nutrients. The advantages of a plant-based diet are numerous and extensive, ranging from lowering the risk of diabetes and heart disease to assisting in healthy weight management and fostering digestive wellness. Beyond its effects on the body, however, a plant-based diet represents an interconnectedness philosophy that acknowledges the close relationship between our personal health, the health of the planet, and the food we eat. Living a plant-based lifestyle respects the delicate ecosystem balance, lessens our ecological impact, and helps ensure future generations have a more sustainable future.

We set out on a path of self-discovery and personal growth as we transition to a plant-based diet, and every meal serves as a chance to nourish our bodies and spirits. We expose ourselves to a world of culinary creativity and sensory delight as we explore new flavors, textures, and possibilities that uplift and inspire us as we venture into the world of plant-based cuisine.

We will go deeper into the ideas and applications of plant-based eating in the pages that follow, providing advice, ideas, and enticing recipes created especially for senior citizens.

Understanding the Benefits of a Plant-Based Diet for Senior Citizens

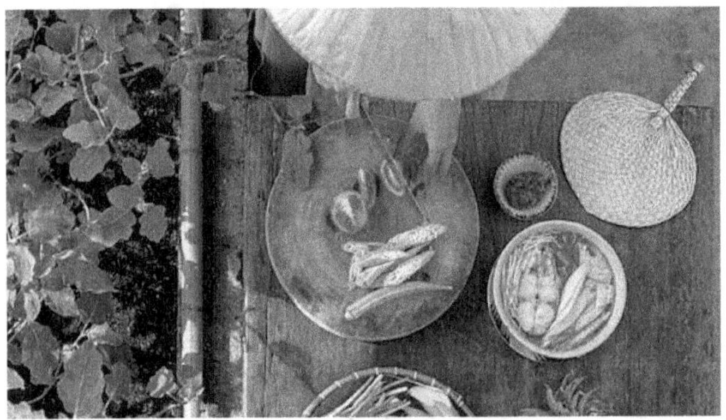

You can benefit greatly from a plant-based diet in many ways that support their health and vitality. Plant-based diets, which are high in fiber, antioxidants, and vital nutrients, help maintain heart health, reduce the risk of chronic illnesses, and encourage appropriate weight management. These foods improve overall health by lowering inflammation and promoting digestive wellness, which builds resistance to age-related illnesses. Diets based primarily on plants also support sustainable living, which recognizes the relationship between environmental stewardship and individual health. Adopting a plant-based diet can help you live longer and more vibrant lives, enabling you to enjoy life to the fullest and live each moment to the fullest.

Nutritional Foundations for Seniors Health on a Plant-Based Diet

It is essential to comprehend the nutritional underpinnings of a plant-based diet if you want to lead the healthiest possible life as a senior. There are many advantages to adopting this lifestyle, but it is critical to meet your individual nutritional needs. Vegetable-based diets are rich in the vitamins, minerals, and antioxidants needed to keep bones strong, aid in digestion, and promote heart health. Make an effort to include a range of nutrient-dense foods in your meals, such as whole grains, legumes, nuts, and leafy greens. As sources of calcium, vitamin D, and vitamin B12 are essential for the health of senior citizens, pay particular attention to what you eat. To ensure nutritional adequacy, take into account adding supplements and fortified plant-based milk substitutes as needed. You create the groundwork for long-term health and vitality in your later years by making a varied and well-balanced plant-based diet your top priority.

Chapter 1: Exploring Key Nutrients and Their Sources

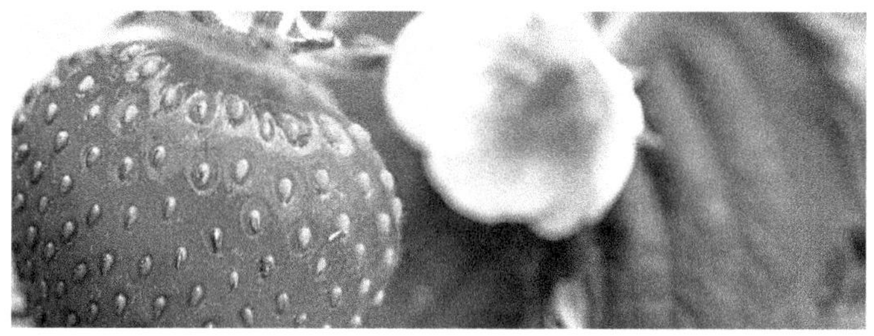

Knowing important nutrients and their sources is essential as you investigate the benefits of a plant-based diet. For healthy bones, calcium is abundant in fortified plant-based milk, tofu, leafy greens like collard greens and kale, and almonds. Fortified plant-based milk, cereals, and sunshine are good sources of vitamin D, which is necessary for the absorption of calcium.

The essential vitamin B12 for healthy nerves can be added to diets by fortifying foods such as nutritional yeast or plant-based milk and cereals. Omega-3 fatty acids are found in flaxseeds, chia seeds, walnuts, and algae-based supplements. These fatty acids are crucial for heart health. Lentils, beans, tofu, spinach, and fortified cereals are good sources of iron, which is necessary for the transportation of oxygen and energy. You can also be sure that you are getting a wide range of vital vitamins, minerals, and antioxidants to support general health and vitality into your senior years by concentrating on a variety of fruits, vegetables, whole grains, and nuts.

Practical Tips for Meeting Nutritional Needs

Take into consideration these useful suggestions designed to support your health and vitality as a senior in order to effectively meet your nutritional needs on a plant-based diet. To begin with, try to vary the foods you eat. Include a wide variety of fruits, vegetables, whole grains, legumes, nuts, and seeds in your meals. This guarantees that you get a wide range of vital vitamins, minerals, and antioxidants. Second, give special attention to foods that are high in nutrients per calorie, such as berries, nuts, and leafy greens. To guarantee sufficient consumption of nutrients like calcium, vitamin D, and vitamin B12—which may be less prevalent in plant-based diets—be wary of fortified foods and supplements. In order to maintain balanced nutrition throughout the day, you should also be mindful of portion sizes and meal frequency. Finally, pay attention to your body's signals and seek the advice of a qualified dietitian or healthcare provider for individualized advice on fulfilling your unique nutritional requirements. You can effectively nourish your body and thrive on a plant-based diet well into your senior years by putting these helpful tips into practice.

Importance of Hydration and Fluid Intake for Aging Bodies

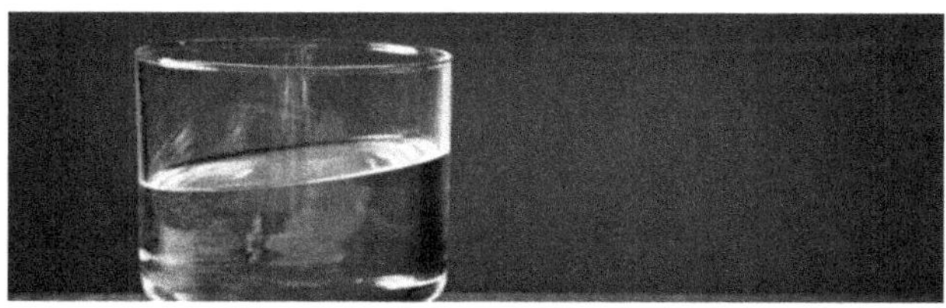

It is impossible to exaggerate the significance of fluid intake and hydration for aging bodies. As I have gotten older, I have realized how important it is to maintain proper hydration for overall health and wellbeing. Because our bodies may become less adept at maintaining fluid balance as we age, staying hydrated is even more important. Maintaining adequate hydration promotes a healthy digestive system, controls body temperature, and facilitates the body's natural flow of nutrients. Conversely, dehydration can result in a number of problems, such as constipation, exhaustion, and UTIs.

I have developed the ability to pay attention to my body's cues and deliberately work to stay hydrated throughout the day. Of course, the best option is water, but for some extra taste and variety, I also like herbal teas, coconut water, and infused water. I have discovered that having a reusable water bottle close by makes it a great reminder to take frequent sips. I also keep an eye out for things like hot weather, physical activity, and certain medications that may raise my fluid requirements.

My daily routine has improved noticeably since I started drinking lots of fluids. My skin appears healthier, I have more energy, and I can handle the rigors of daily life better. I am being proactive in supporting my aging body and making sure I can keep living life to the fullest for years to come by making hydration a priority.

Smart Shopping and Meal Planning Strategies

For senior citizens such as yourself, a little advance planning goes a long way toward guaranteeing that you always have wholesome and delectable meals on hand. Make a list of your favorite plant-based staples that meet your nutritional needs, such as fruits, vegetables, whole grains, legumes, nuts, and seeds. Make a list of everything you already own before you go to the grocery store to help you avoid making unnecessary purchases.

When you shop, give priority to seasonal and fresh produce; for convenience and adaptability, consider frozen and canned options as well. Beans, lentils, and whole grains are affordable options that you can find in the bulk section or during sales. To save costs and cut down on the number of times you have to visit the store, think about buying things in bigger quantities.

Make time to plan your meals once you are back at home. For the upcoming week, pick a few recipes that you want to try from your plant-based cookbook, making sure to plan for any leftovers or ingredients that you can use in different ways. To have large quantities of grains, beans, or soups on hand for quick and simple meals all week, think about batch cooking them.

Last but not least, remember to properly store your groceries to extend their shelf life and freshness. Dry goods should be kept out of direct sunlight in a cool, dry place; perishables, such as fruits and vegetables, should be kept in the refrigerator. With these clever shopping and meal planning tips, you will be ready to fuel your body with wholesome, tasty plant-based meals every day.

Guide to Selecting Fresh, Seasonal Produce

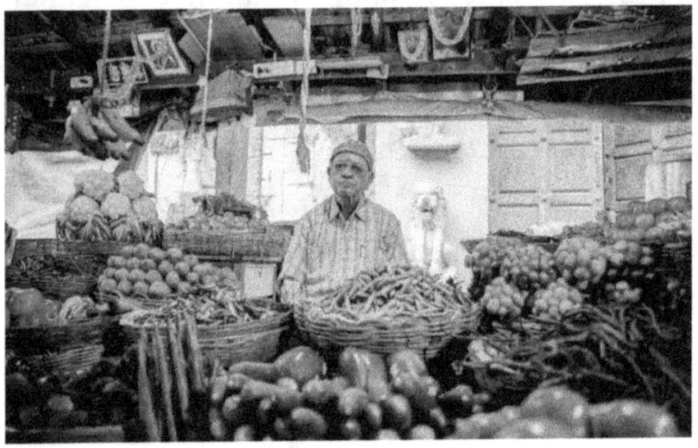

I have discovered that a little knowledge goes a long way toward ensuring that I bring home the best fruits and vegetables when it comes to choosing fresh, in-season produce. I have developed the habit of beginning by looking for freshness indicators, such as vivid colors, firm textures, and crisp leaves, which denote the best quality in the produce. I take my time looking over each item at the farmers' market or grocery store, gently squeezing fruits to determine their ripeness and smelling herbs to determine their aroma.

I have also developed an awareness of the seasonal changes and realized that fruits and vegetables are typically at their healthiest and tastiest when they are in season. Summer brings me juicy berries, luscious tomatoes, and crunchy cucumbers; fall brings me the earthy sweetness of pumpkins, apples, and squash. Selecting in-season produce not only results in better flavor and quality, but it also helps local farmers and lowers my carbon footprint.

I place a high value on choosing organic produce whenever I can since it is grown without the use of artificial fertilizers or pesticides, and it is also fresher and in season. Even though organic products could cost a little more, I see them as an investment in both the environment and my health.

Tips for Reading Food Labels and Adapting Recipes

Remember the following advice when modifying recipes and reading food labels: Look through ingredient lists for any hidden allergens or additives. Aim for ingredients that are whole and have undergone minimal processing; steer clear of products with long, obscure names.

Be mindful of serving sizes and the amount of nutrients in each serving. Try substituting plant-based ingredients for meat, such as tofu or beans, and eggs, such as applesauce or flaxseed, when modifying recipes.

Use your imagination and do not be scared to modify recipes to fit your dietary requirements and tastes. You can become an expert at reading labels and modifying recipes to suit your plant-based diet with a little practice.

Budget-Friendly Shopping and Meal Planning

Several strategies exist for frugal shopping and meal planning that allow you to enjoy nutrient-dense plant-based meals without breaking the bank. Make a list of the most reasonably priced staples you can find, such as rice, pasta, beans, lentils, oats, and frozen fruits and vegetables. To save money on these things, look for deals, discounts, and bulk purchasing options. Additionally, you might be able to find better deals on fresh produce at ethnic grocery stores or local farmers' markets.

When organizing your meals, give special attention to easy, affordable recipes that make use of inexpensive or readily available ingredients. By enabling you to prepare large amounts of food at once and portion it out for multiple meals throughout the week, batch cooking and meal prepping can also help you save time and money.

Remember to use your imagination when preparing leftovers and repurposing ingredients to cut down on waste. For instance, you can make fried rice or stir-fry with leftover rice, and you can use soups or stews with wilted vegetables.

You can enjoy tasty and nourishing plant-based meals without going over budget by using these frugal shopping and meal planning tips.

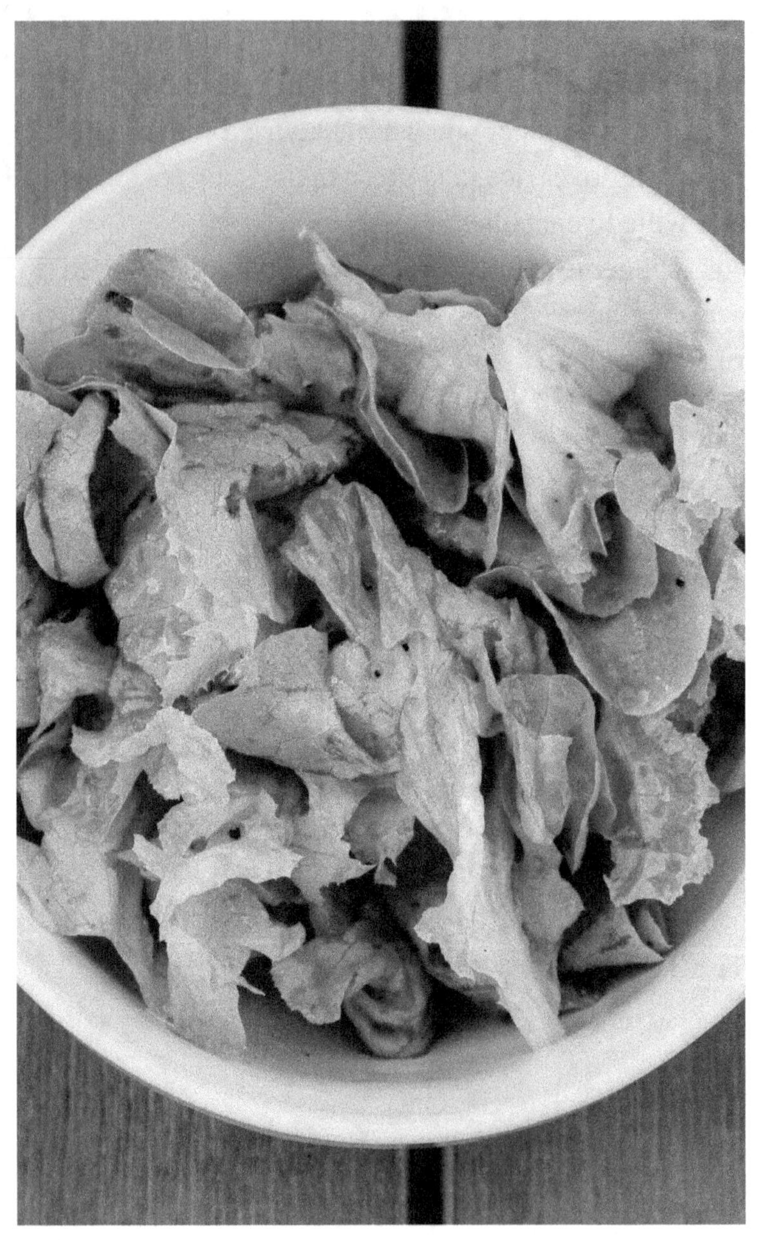

Chapter 2: Cooking Techniques and Kitchen Adaptations for Seniors

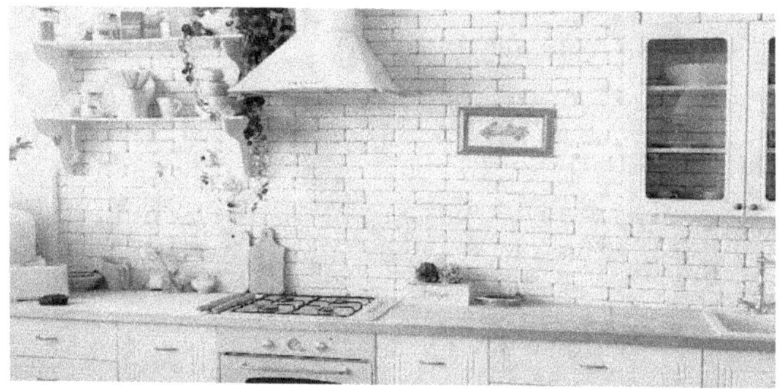

Meal preparation can be made more enjoyable and easier with the right cooking techniques and kitchen adaptations designed for seniors like you. To minimize bending or stretching, start by arranging your kitchen so that everything is easily accessible. Invest in jar openers, lightweight cookware, easy-grip utensils, and other ergonomic kitchen appliances made with senior citizens in mind.

When it comes to cooking, choose methods that are easy to understand and require little work. One-pot cooking, steaming, and stir-frying are all excellent choices for simple and quick meals. To save time and effort, think about utilizing pre-cut or pre-packaged ingredients. You can also ask family members or caregivers to assist with meal preparation.

Never be scared to use your imagination and try out novel flavors and ingredients. Cooking is a rewarding and enjoyable activity, and there are plenty of plant-based recipes to try. You can enjoy tasty and nourishing meals well into your senior years with a few easy changes to your kitchen and cooking habits.

Easy and Safe Cooking Methods for Aging Hands and Bodies

The two most important considerations when cooking with aging hands and bodies are safety and ease. Choose to cook with techniques that are easy on your hands and do not take much work. Pressure cookers and crockpots are great options for slow cooking because they require little to no hands-on time to prepare delicious meals. Take extra care when handling knives and other sharp objects to prevent mishaps. Use cutting boards with non-slip grips, put on knife guards, and think about buying ergonomic utensils.

If you find it difficult to stand for extended periods of time, think about getting a good stool or chair to help you while you cook. As an alternative, search for recipes that call for little time spent standing, like one-pot dishes or recipes that can be made while seated.

Lastly, never be afraid to ask for assistance when you need it. Ask your loved ones, caregivers, or friends for help with meal preparation or other household chores that might be too much for you to handle alone. Long into your golden years, you can still enjoy cooking and creating delectable meals by putting safety and convenience first in the kitchen.

Essential Kitchen Tools and Appliances

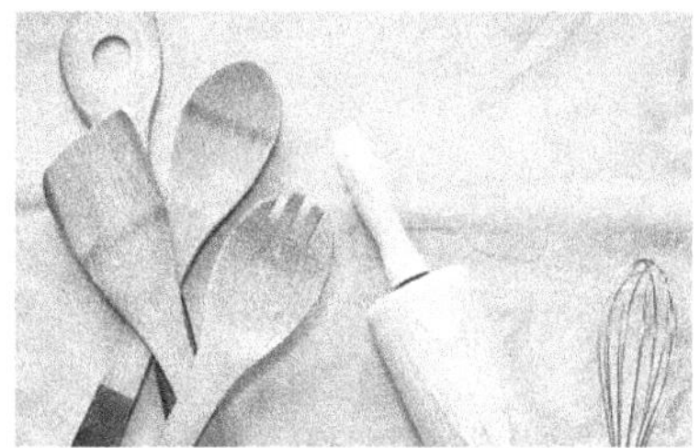

When it comes to setting up your kitchen for easy and efficient cooking, having the right tools and appliances can make all the difference. Here are some essential items to consider:

- **Ergonomic Utensils:** Invest in utensils with comfortable, easy-to-grip handles to minimize strain on your hands and wrists.

- **Non-Slip Cutting Board:** Choose a cutting board with a non-slip surface to provide stability and prevent accidents while chopping and slicing.

- **Lightweight Cookware:** Opt for pots and pans made from lightweight materials such as aluminum or stainless steel to make lifting and maneuvering easier.

- **Electric Can Opener:** A handy electric can opener eliminates the need for manual twisting and can be operated with the touch of a button.

- **Jar Opener:** Look for a jar opener with a nonslip grip or adjustable design to help you easily open stubborn lids.

- **Blender or Food Processor:** These versatile appliances can be used to puree soups, blend smoothies, and chop vegetables with ease.

- **Slow Cooker or Crockpot:** Perfect for hands-off cooking, a slow cooker allows you to prepare delicious meals with minimal effort.

- **Microwave:** A microwave oven is invaluable for quickly reheating leftovers, steaming vegetables, and cooking convenience foods.

- **Electric Kettle:** Boil water in minutes for tea, coffee, or cooking with the convenience of an electric kettle.

- **Kitchen Stool or Chair:** Consider keeping a sturdy stool or chair nearby to provide support and rest during meal preparation. A soft chair will be recommended.

With these essential kitchen tools and appliances on hand, you'll be well-equipped to tackle any recipe with ease and confidence.

Strategies for Overcoming Common Kitchen Challenges

When faced with typical kitchen obstacles, it is critical to tackle them creatively and adaptably. Here are some methods to get past these challenges:

- **Limited Mobility:** If you have trouble moving around the kitchen due to mobility issues, think about setting up your workspace effectively to reduce the amount of movement that is necessary. Store items that are frequently used close to hand and use reachers or grabbers with long handles to reach higher shelves.

- **Vision Impairments:** To make cooking easier for those with vision impairments, use tactile cues and contrasting colors. Make use of cutting boards and utensils with high contrast, and make sure to label spices and ingredients with legible labels. Use kitchen appliances that have tactile indicators, like Braille markings or raised dots.

- **Fatigue:** If fatigue sets in during meal preparation, pace yourself and take breaks as needed. Consider breaking down tasks into smaller, manageable steps and enlist the help of family members or caregivers when necessary. Alternatively, explore cooking methods that require less hands-on time, such as slow cooking or batch cooking.

- **Arthritis or Joint Pain:** For individuals with arthritis or joint pain, choose kitchen tools and appliances with ergonomic handles and easy-grip designs. Use adaptive aids such as jar openers, electric can openers, and cutting boards with stabilizing grips to minimize strain on arthritic joints.

- **Memory Loss or Cognitive Impairment:** To navigate kitchen tasks with memory loss or cognitive impairment, create a visual checklist or step-by-step guide for meal preparation. Keep cooking instructions simple and repetitive, and consider using color-coded labels or pictures to aid in ingredient recognition.

By implementing these strategies and making small adjustments to your kitchen routine, you can overcome common challenges and continue to enjoy cooking and meal preparation with ease and confidence.

Mindful Eating Guide for Seniors

"Picture this: you're seated at the table, surrounded by tantalizing aromas and vibrant colors. But before you dig in, take a moment to breathe. Mindful eating isn't just about what's on your plate—it's about savoring every bite, engaging your senses, and truly appreciating the nourishment before you. For seniors, mindful eating can improve digestion, prevent overeating, and enhance overall well-being. Ready to embark on this journey? Order your copy of the mindful eating guide today and enjoy great benefits!! Scan this code and get your copy now!!

Chapter 3: Energizing Breakfast Ideas for Senior Vitality

Vibrant Berry Smoothie Bowl

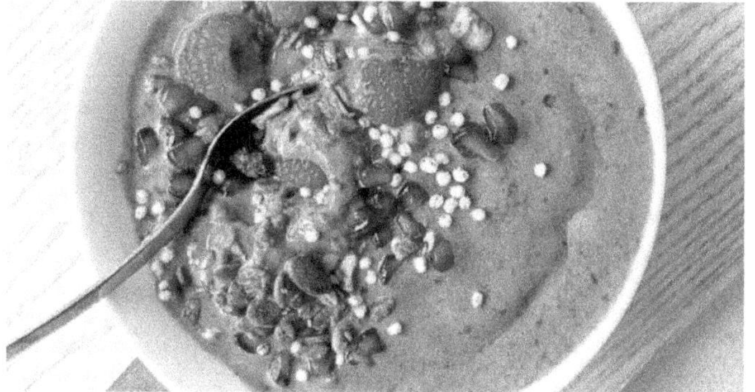

This colorful smoothie bowl of berries will give you a nutritional and flavorful boost to start the day.

Ingredients: Almond milk, chia seeds, granola, banana, spinach, mixed berries (strawberries, blueberries, raspberries), and sliced almonds.

Instructions for Preparation: Blend spinach, almond milk, banana, and mixed berries until smooth. Pour into a bowl and top with chia seeds, granola, and sliced almonds.

Nutritional Information: This smoothie bowl is a great way to start the day because it is full of fiber, vitamins, and minerals, as well as antioxidants.

Protein-Packed Tofu Scramble

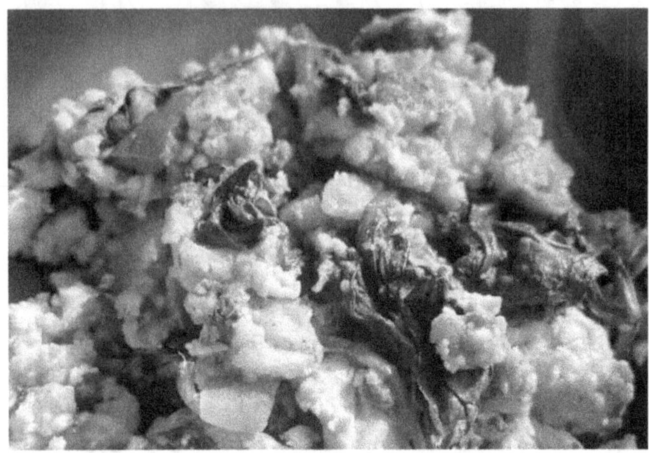

A tasty and filling substitute for traditional scrambled eggs, this protein-rich tofu scramble will fuel your morning.

Ingredients: nutritional yeast, turmeric, garlic powder, bell peppers, onions, spinach, and firm tofu.

Instructions for Preparation: Crumble the tofu into a skillet and add the onions, bell peppers, and spinach. Add nutritional yeast, garlic powder, turmeric, salt, and pepper for seasoning.

Nutritional Information: Packed with vitamins, minerals, and plant-based protein, this tofu scramble promotes muscle health and gives you sustained energy.

Hearty Oatmeal with Fruit and Nuts

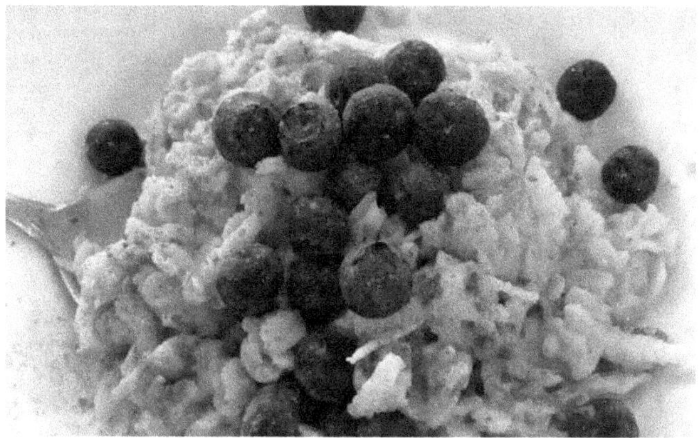

Introduction: Start your morning with a cozy bowl of thick oatmeal sprinkled with almonds and fresh fruit.

Ingredients: Almond milk, cinnamon, maple syrup, rolled oats, bananas, apples, walnuts, and raisins.

Instructions for Preparation: Cook rolled oats in almond milk, maple syrup, and cinnamon until they become creamy. Top with chopped walnuts, raisins, diced apples, and banana slices.

Nutritional Information: Packed full of fiber, protein, and good fats, this bowl of oatmeal gives you long-lasting energy and supports heart health.

The Superfood Acai Bowl

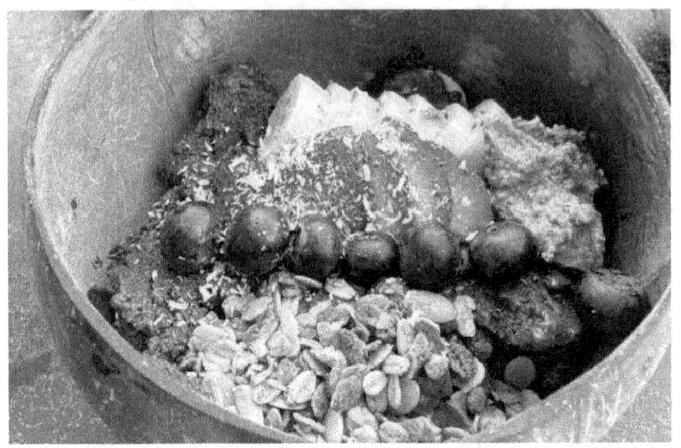

Introduction: Treat yourself to a breakfast full of superfoods with this hydrating acai bowl, which is bursting with vital nutrients and antioxidants.

Ingredients: Almond milk, granola, hemp seeds, banana, frozen acai puree, and mixed berries.

Instructions for Preparation: Blend almond milk, banana, mixed berries, and acai puree until smooth. Transfer into a bowl and garnish with hemp seeds, coconut flakes, and granola.

Nutritional Information: Packed with vitamins, omega-3 fatty acids, and antioxidants, this acai bowl helps maintain healthy brain and immune systems.

Whole Grain Toast with Avocado and Tomato

Introduction: Try this wholesome whole grain toast with creamy avocado and juicy tomato slices for a simple yet satisfying meal.

Ingredients: red pepper flakes, olive oil, lemon juice, avocado, whole grain bread, and tomatoes.

Instructions for Preparation: Toast the whole grain bread, then top with sliced tomatoes, mashed avocado, lemon juice, olive oil, and a pinch of salt, pepper, and red pepper flakes.

Nutritional Information: Packed with vitamins, fiber, and good fats, this toast offers a satisfying and well-balanced way to start the day.

Quinoa Breakfast Bowl with Mixed Fruit

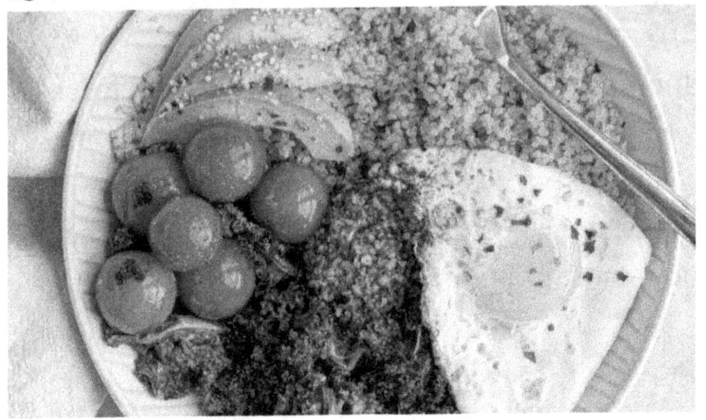

For a filling and healthy breakfast, start your day with a protein-rich quinoa bowl topped with a mix of fresh fruit.

Ingredients: Quinoa, maple syrup, almond milk, vanilla extract, almond slices, mixed fruit (kiwis, mangoes, and berries).

Steps for Preparation: Cook quinoa in almond milk with vanilla extract until it becomes fluffy. Present the dish in a bowl and garnish with almond slices, mixed fruit, and a maple syrup drizzle. You can add egg if desired.

Nutritious Information: Quinoa is a complete protein and, when paired with fresh fruit, offers a well-balanced combination of fiber, carbohydrates, vitamins, and minerals to support long-term energy.

Chia Seed Pudding with Coconut and Berries

First up, treat yourself to a delicious breakfast treat of rich, creamy, coconut-flavored chia seed pudding topped with a luscious burst of fresh berries.

Ingredients: Chia seeds, coconut milk, maple syrup, vanilla extract, shredded coconut, mixed berries.

Instructions for Preparation: Combine coconut milk, vanilla extract, and chia seeds. Refrigerate until the mixture thickens. Garnish with mixed berries and shredded coconut.

Nutritional Information: Mixed berries add vitamins and antioxidants, and chia seeds, which are high in omega-3 fatty acids, when combined with coconut milk, offer a source of fiber and healthy fats.

Banana Walnut Pancakes

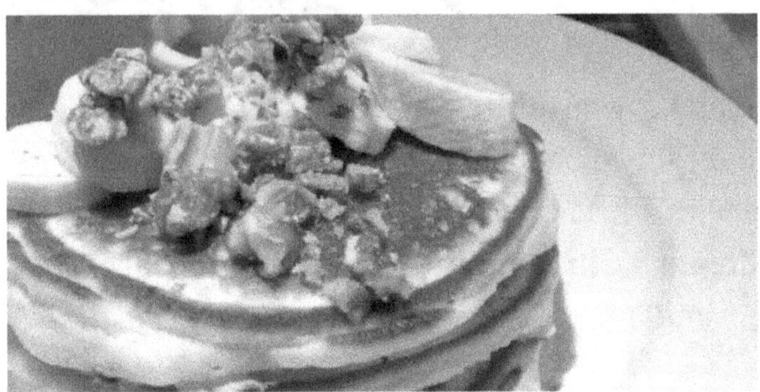

Introduction: For a satisfying and nutrient-dense breakfast option, savor fluffy and hearty banana walnut pancakes made with whole grain flour. Ingredients include walnuts, almond milk, ripe bananas, baking powder, cinnamon, and maple syrup.

Instructions for Preparation: Combine almond milk, chopped walnuts, cinnamon, baking powder, and mashed bananas with whole grain flour. In a nonstick skillet, cook pancakes until golden brown. Drizzle with maple syrup and serve.

Nutritional Information: Packed with fiber, potassium, and good fats from walnuts and bananas, these pancakes make a hearty and filling breakfast option.

Spinach and Mushroom Breakfast Burrito

Start your day off right with a tasty breakfast burrito made with spinach, mushrooms, and tofu scramble that is packed full of protein and tasty vegetables.

Ingredients: salsa, firm tofu, nutritional yeast, garlic powder, onions, mushrooms, and spinach with whole wheat tortillas.

Preparation Instructions: Cook firm tofu with onions, mushrooms, and spinach.
Add some turmeric, garlic powder, and nutritional yeast for seasoning. Top whole wheat tortillas with salsa and spoon on tofu scramble. Roll up and serve.

Nutritional Information: Packed with protein, vitamins, and minerals from tofu, spinach, and mushrooms, this breakfast burrito is a filling and healthy way to start the day.

Coconut Yogurt Parfait with Tropical Fruit

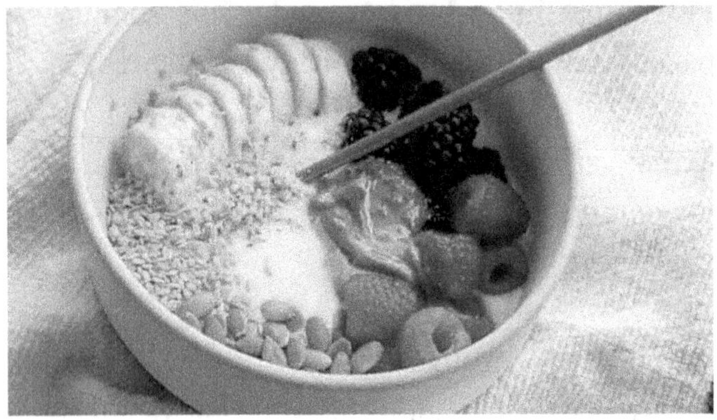

Introduction: For a cool and filling breakfast, indulge in a coconut yogurt parfait with a tropical flair, composed of layers of creamy yogurt, ripe tropical fruit, and crunchy granola.

Ingredients: granola, shredded coconut, honey or agave syrup, mango, pineapple, and kiwi.

Instructions for Preparation: Arrange diced mango, pineapple, and kiwi in a glass or bowl with coconut yogurt. Top with granola, shredded coconut, and a drizzle of honey or agave syrup.

Nutritional Information: This parfait is a tasty and filling breakfast choice because coconut yogurt offers probiotics for gut health and tropical fruit provides a dose of vitamins, minerals, and antioxidants.

Hearty Whole Grain Breakfasts

These substantial whole grain breakfasts will fuel you up and satisfy you all day. They are full of fiber, vitamins, and minerals.

Whole Grain Pancakes with Mixed Berries:

For a delightful breakfast, treat yourself to fluffy whole grain pancakes topped with a vibrant assortment of mixed berries.

Ingredients: baking powder, banana, mixed berries, maple syrup, whole wheat flour, and almond milk.

Instructions for Preparation: Blend almond milk, mashed banana, and whole wheat flour until smooth. In a nonstick skillet, cook pancakes until golden brown. Drizzle with maple syrup and garnish with a mixture of berries.

Nutritional Information: Packed with vitamins, fiber, and antioxidants, these pancakes make a satisfying and healthy breakfast.

Quinoa Breakfast Bowl with Fruit and Nuts:

Introduction: For a filling and nutritious breakfast, start your day with a protein-rich quinoa bowl topped with crunchy nuts and fresh fruit.

Quinoa, apples, bananas, walnuts, raisins, cinnamon, maple syrup, and almond milk are among the ingredients.

Instructions for Preparation: Cook quinoa until fluffy by adding almond milk, cinnamon, and maple syrup. Top with chopped walnuts, raisins, diced apples, and banana slices.

Nutritional Information: Packed with vital nutrients, fiber, and protein, this breakfast bowl promotes general health and wellbeing.

Whole Grain Toast with Avocado and Tomato:

For a hearty breakfast option, keep things simple but satisfying with this nutrient-dense whole grain toast topped with creamy avocado and juicy tomato slices.

Ingredients: red pepper flakes, olive oil, lemon juice, avocado, whole grain bread, and tomatoes.

Instructions for Preparation: Toast the whole grain bread, then top with sliced tomatoes, mashed avocado, lemon juice, olive oil, and a pinch of salt, pepper, and red pepper flakes.

Nutritional Information: Packed with vitamins, minerals, and healthy fats, this avocado toast offers a satisfying and well-balanced way to start the day.

Oatmeal with Chia Seeds and Fresh Fruit:

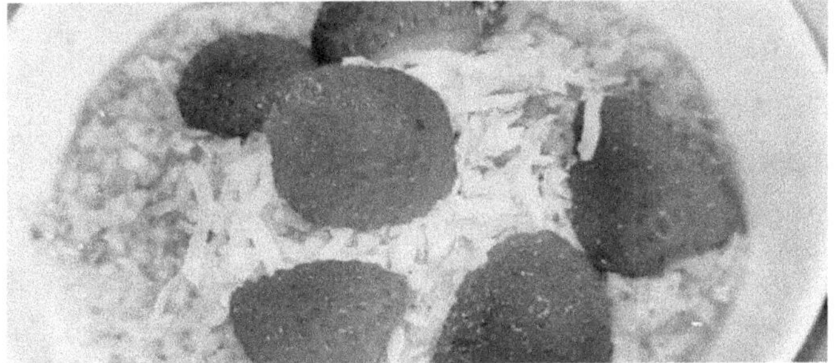

For a hearty and satisfying breakfast, start your morning with a cozy bowl of oatmeal topped with a variety of fresh fruit and nutrient-dense chia seeds.

Almond milk, chia seeds, honey, maple syrup, sliced banana, rolled oats, mixed berries, and almonds are the ingredients.

Preparation Instructions: Cook rolled oats with almond milk until creamy. Add the chia seeds and use honey or maple syrup to sweeten. Add almonds, sliced banana, and mixed berries on top.

Nutritional Information: Packed with antioxidants, omega-3 fatty acids, and fiber, this oatmeal bowl makes a filling and healthy breakfast.

Quinoa Breakfast Bowl with Mixed Berries and Almonds:

Fill up on protein, fiber, and antioxidants with a filling and healthy quinoa breakfast bowl to start your day.

The ingredients include quinoa, almond milk, cinnamon, maple syrup, sliced almonds, and a mixture of berries (strawberries, blueberries, and raspberries).

Preparation Instructions: Prepare the quinoa by rinsing it well and cooking it as directed on the package, substituting almond milk for water to make it creamier. After the quinoa is cooked, place it in a bowl and garnish with sliced almonds, mixed berries, cinnamon, and maple syrup.

Nutritional Details: Packed full of vital vitamins and minerals, this quinoa breakfast bowl offers a well-balanced combination of healthy fats, carbohydrates, and protein. Quinoa provides a complete protein source, and almonds and berries provide heart-healthy fats and antioxidants.

With vital nutrients and energy for maximum health and vitality, these substantial whole grain breakfasts provide seniors with a tasty and nourishing way to start their day. Take pleasure in experimenting with various pairings and adding these healthful meals to your regular rotation!

Fruit-Based Options for Morning Energy

Mango Coconut Smoothie Bowl:

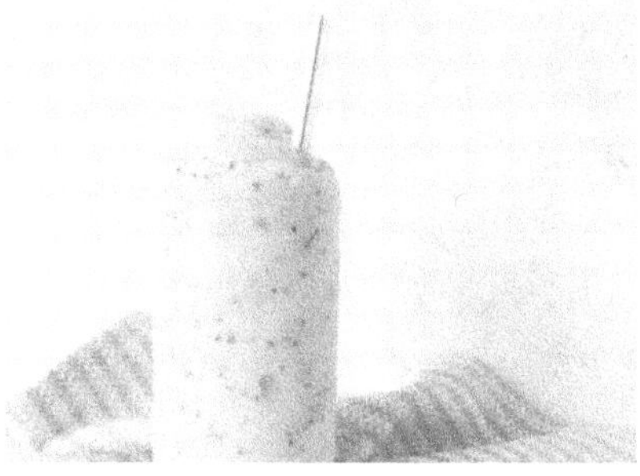

Energize your morning with this tropical delight! Bursting with the goodness of mango and coconut, this smoothie bowl will leave you feeling refreshed and ready to tackle the day ahead.

Ingredients: Ripe mango, coconut milk, banana, shredded coconut, granola, chia seeds.

Instructions for Preparation: Blend the banana, coconut milk, and mango until smooth. Transfer into a bowl, then garnish with granola, chia seeds, and shredded coconut for extra nutrition and texture.

Nutritional Information: The mango, coconut, and chia seeds in this smoothie bowl provide a good source of healthy fats, fiber, and vitamin C. It gives you a nourishing and revitalizing start to the day.

Berry Breakfast Parfait:

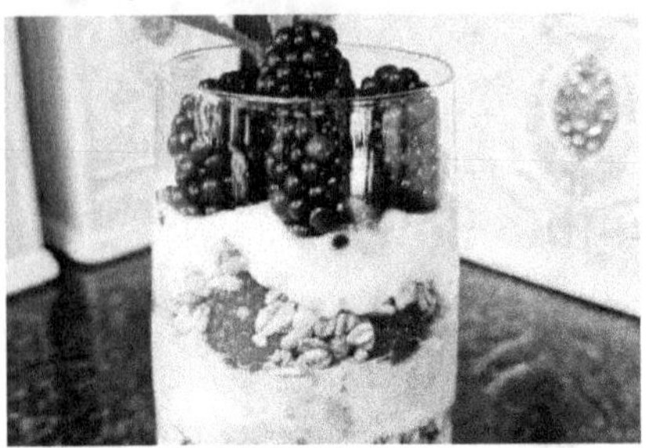

Treat yourself to a vibrant and delicious berry breakfast parfait! It is a delicious way to start the day, layered with crunchy granola, creamy yogurt, and juicy berries.

Ingredients: Granola, plant-based yogurt, mixed berries (strawberries, blueberries, raspberries), and optional honey or maple syrup.

Preparation Instructions: In a glass or bowl, alternate layers of berries, yogurt, and granola. Drizzle with honey or maple syrup if desired. Repeat layers until the glass or bowl is filled. Enjoy the burst of flavors and textures!

Nutritional Information: This parfait is packed with antioxidants, probiotics, and fiber from the berries, yogurt, and granola. It provides a balanced mix of carbohydrates, protein, and fats to fuel your morning.

Pineapple Coconut Chia Pudding:

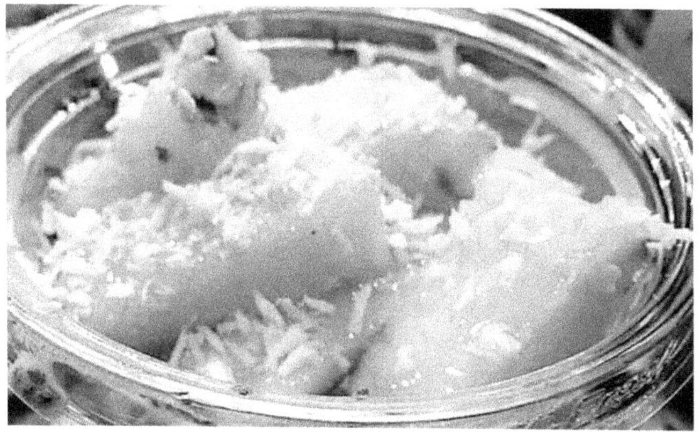

Transport yourself to a tropical paradise with this pineapple coconut chia pudding! Creamy, satisfying, and packed with nutrients, it's the perfect way to start your day on a refreshing note.

Ingredients: Chia seeds, coconut milk, pineapple chunks, shredded coconut, maple syrup.

Preparation Instructions: Mix chia seeds, coconut milk, and maple syrup in a bowl. Let it sit in the refrigerator for at least 4 hours or overnight until thickened. Layer with pineapple chunks and shredded coconut before serving.

Nutritional Information: This chia pudding is rich in omega-3 fatty acids, fiber, and vitamins from the chia seeds and coconut milk. Pineapple adds a burst of vitamin C and sweetness to the dish.

Apple Cinnamon Oatmeal:

Warm up your morning with this comforting apple cinnamon oatmeal! Packed with fiber, protein, and natural sweetness, it's a classic breakfast option that never disappoints.

Ingredients: Rolled oats, almond milk, apple, cinnamon, maple syrup, chopped nuts (optional).

Preparation Instructions: Cook oats with almond milk, chopped apple, cinnamon, and maple syrup until creamy. Top with chopped nuts for added crunch and protein. Serve warm and enjoy!

Nutritional Information: This oatmeal provides a balanced mix of complex carbohydrates, fiber, and protein from the oats, apple, and nuts. It's a filling and nourishing breakfast choice.

Banana Berry Breakfast Wrap:

Shake up your morning routine with this fun and flavorful banana berry breakfast wrap! Wrapped in a whole grain tortilla, it's a convenient and portable option for busy mornings.

Ingredients: Whole grain tortilla, almond butter, banana, mixed berries, hemp seeds.

Preparation Instructions: Spread almond butter on a tortilla and layer with sliced banana, mixed berries, and hemp seeds. Roll up the tortilla tightly and slice into bite-sized pieces or enjoy as a wrap.

Nutritional Information: This breakfast wrap offers a balance of carbohydrates, healthy fats, and protein from the whole grain tortilla, almond butter, fruit, and hemp seeds. It's a satisfying and energizing option to fuel your morning activities.

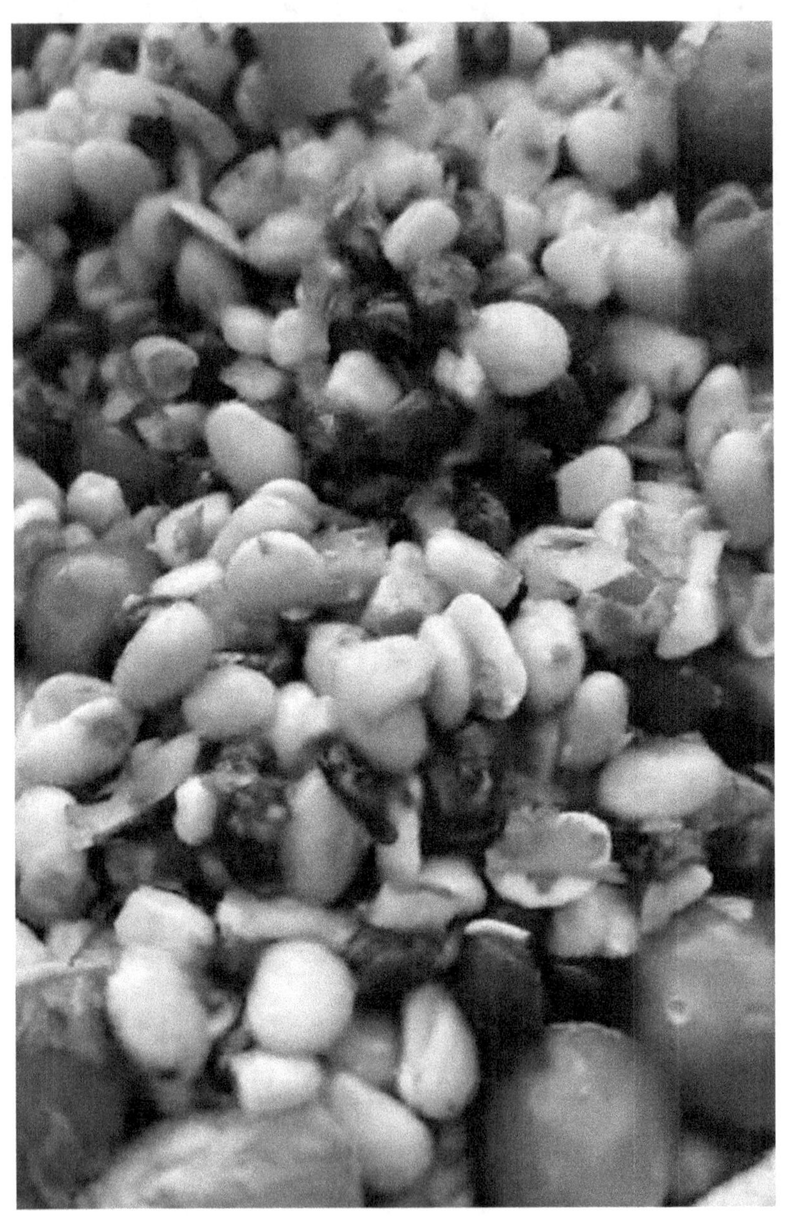

Chapter 4: Wholesome Lunches for Sustained Senior Wellness

Quinoa Salad with Roasted Vegetables:

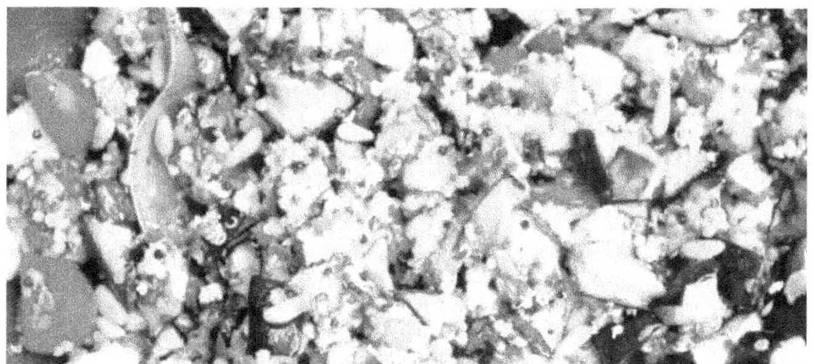

Nourish your body with this vibrant and nutrient-rich quinoa salad, packed with roasted vegetables for a satisfying and wholesome lunch option.

INGREDIENTS

- One cup cooked quinoa or ⅓ cup uncooked quinoa that has been rinsed
- Diced one small eggplant, about ¾ pound in size.
- One small zucchini, chopped
- One tiny yellow squash (or other type of zucchini), chopped
- Three to four tablespoons, divided between
- Sea salt and recently ground black pepper

- To taste, add 1 ½ to 2 tablespoons of lemon juice (about 1 medium lemon).
- One minced or pressed garlic clove
- Quarter any larger tomatoes, or half a cup of grape tomatoes.
- two tablespoons of freshly chopped basil leaves
- two tsp finely chopped mint leaves
- Two tablespoons of toasted pine nuts
- Crumbled feta on top, if desired

INSTRUCTIONS

- Adjust oven racks to upper and lower thirds and preheat to 425 degrees Fahrenheit. Put parchment paper on two large, rimmed baking sheets.
- Split the yellow squash, zucchini, and eggplant between the two baking sheets. Pour in one tablespoon of olive oil and mix. If needed, add a little bit more; you only need to coat the veggies lightly. Add a dash of pepper and salt. Roast for 20 to 30 minutes, or until the vegetables are soft and starting to brown. After roasting, set the veggies aside to cool.
- To cook the quinoa, put the raw quinoa in a small saucepan with ⅔ cup water. Over

medium-high heat, bring to a boil; after that, cover and turn down the heat. After about 15 minutes of simmering until the water is absorbed, turn off the heat and leave the quinoa covered to steam for five minutes. Take off the lid, use a fork to fluff the quinoa, and set it aside.

- To toast the pine nuts, place them in a small skillet over medium heat and stir them around frequently. Cook for 5 to 10 minutes, or until they start to turn lightly golden and smell fragrant. To prevent them from burning, be sure to keep an eye on them. To cool, transfer to a bowl.

- Whisk the garlic and lemon juice together in a large serving bowl. To emulsify the mixture, slowly pour in the remaining 2 tablespoons of olive oil while whisking continuously. Gently stir in the quinoa, tomatoes, roasted vegetables, basil, mint, and pine nuts. Add plenty of salt, pepper, and, if desired, another squeeze of lemon to season. If desired, garnish with crumbled feta.

Calories Count: Approximately 300-350 calories per serving.

Prep Time: 30 minutes.

Chickpea and Avocado Wrap:

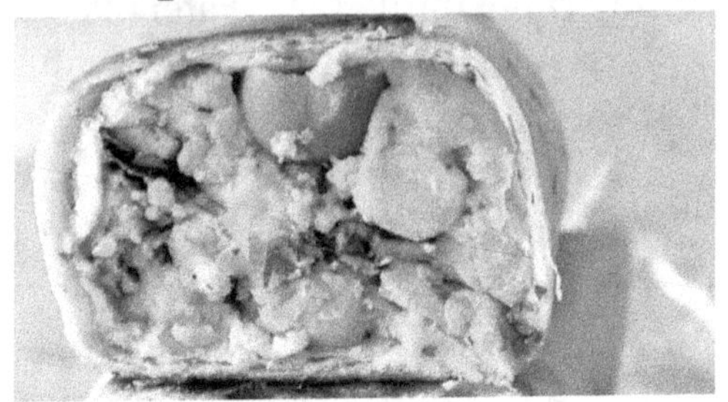

Enjoy a protein-packed and flavorful lunch with this chickpea and avocado wrap, filled with creamy avocado, tangy hummus, and crunchy veggies.

Preparation Method: Mash chickpeas with avocado, lemon juice, salt, and pepper to create a creamy filling. Spread hummus onto a whole grain tortilla, top with the chickpea-avocado mixture, sliced cucumber, shredded carrots, and baby spinach. Roll up the tortilla tightly and slice into halves or thirds.

Ingredients: Chickpeas, avocado, lemon juice, salt, pepper, whole grain tortilla, hummus, cucumber, carrots, baby spinach.

Step 1: Place half of the chickpeas, half of the parsley, and half of the mint in a blender (or, if you have an immersion blender, a bowl). An additional bit of work would be required if you decided to mash the chickpeas by hand.

Step 2: Include the sesame seeds, garlic, olive oil, lemon juice, and chili powder. Mash or blend until extremely smooth.

Step 3: When this mixture is ready, add the remaining chickpeas.

Step 4: Spoon half of this mixture onto a small tortilla, then top with avocado, sliced olives, and the remaining parsley and mint. Make a burrito-like fold.

Step 5: Toast the wrap, starting with the open side to seal, in a nonstick pan. After that, turn over and toast the other side as well.

Calories Count: Approximately 350-400 calories per serving.

Prep Time: 15 minutes.

Sweet Potato and Black Bean Buddha Bowl

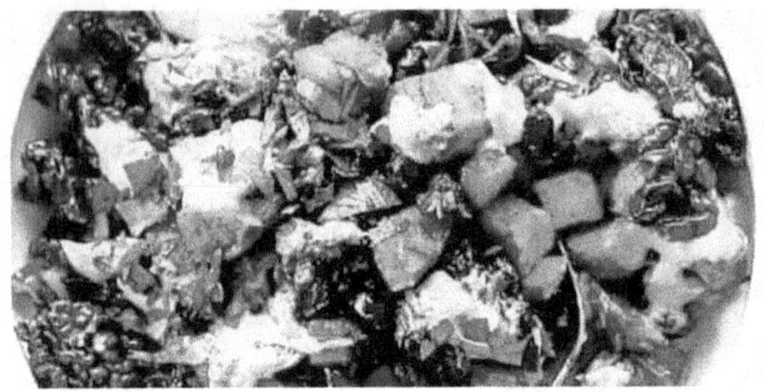

Treat yourself to a nourishing Buddha bowl featuring roasted sweet potatoes, black beans, and a variety of colorful veggies, all served over a bed of fluffy quinoa.

Ingredients: Sweet potatoes, black beans, quinoa, avocado, cherry tomatoes, kale, tahini dressing, olive oil, garlic powder.

Preparation Instructions:

Step 1: To roast sweet potatoes, cut them into small cubes, coat them with olive oil, season with salt, pepper, chili powder, and garlic powder, and toss again. After arranging the potatoes in a single layer on a baking sheet, roast them at 425 degrees Fahrenheit for 25 minutes. according to the recipe card that is attached.

Step 2: Cook the black beans by sautéing th e garlic, onions, and peppers in a skillet with a little oil added.

To bring out all of the flavor, season, add the black beans, and cook for a few minutes. Set aside.

Step 3: Sauté the kale: In a large skillet over medium heat, add the garlic and olive oil. Add the sliced kale (you can also use baby spinach in this recipe), and cook until the kale is wilted. roughly three to four minutes.

Blend the sauce. In a high-speed blender, add all the sauce ingredients and blend until smooth.

Step 4: Create your bowl of Buddha. In a bowl, combine some of the cooked black beans, roasted sweet potatoes, and sautéed greens. Drizzle with some of the creamy sauce, and serve!

Calories Count: Approximately 400-450 calories per serving.

Prep Time: 45 minutes.

Mushroom and Lentil Soup:

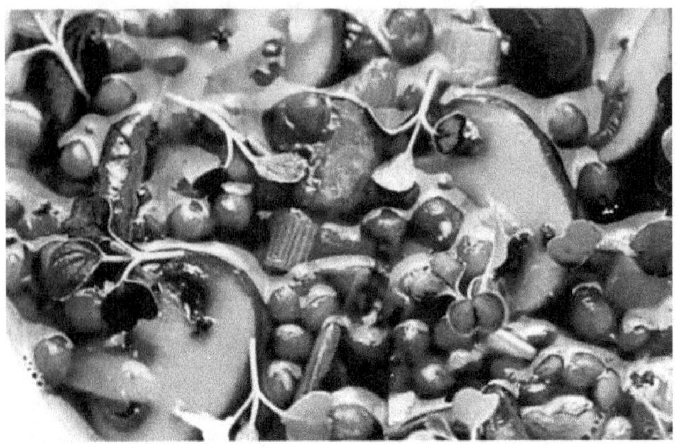

Warm up with a satisfying and filling soup made with lentils, which are high in fiber, savory mushrooms, and fragrant herbs and spices.

Preparation Method:

Step 1: Sauté onions, garlic, and celery in a pot until softened.

Step 2: Include the diced tomatoes, thyme, bay leaves, cooked lentils, and sliced mushrooms.

Step 3: Simmer the soup until the flavors combine and it becomes slightly thicker. Garnish with freshly chopped parsley and serve warm.

Ingredients: Lentils, mushrooms, onion, garlic, celery, vegetable broth, diced tomatoes, thyme, bay leaves, parsley.

Calories Count: Approximately 250-300 calories per serving.

Prep Time: 40 minutes.

Tofu Stir-Fry with Brown Rice

This tofu stir-fry, loaded with vibrant vegetables and served over nutty brown rice, makes a filling and well-balanced lunch option.

Preparation Method:

Step 1: Tofu should be pressed to remove extra moisture before being cut into cubes and stir-fried in a pan until golden brown.

Step 2: Add the garlic, ginger, and soy sauce to a separate pan and sauté mixed vegetables (like bell peppers, broccoli, carrots, and snap peas) until they are crisp-tender.

Step 3: Top cooked brown rice with tofu and veggies, and sprinkle with sesame seeds and green onions.

Ingredients: Tofu, mixed vegetables, garlic, ginger, soy sauce, brown rice, green onions, sesame seeds.

Calories Count: Approximately 350-400 calories per serving.

Prep Time: 30 minutes.

Chickpea Salad Sandwich:

This chickpea salad sandwich, stuffed with crunchy veggies, tart lemon-dill dressing, and creamy mashed chickpeas, makes a filling and high-protein lunch.

Preparation Instructions:

Step 1: Chickpeas should be mashed with lemon juice, Dijon mustard, dill, salt, and pepper for preparation.

Step 2: Add the bell pepper, red onion, and diced celery. Spread the whole grain bread slices with the chickpea salad, top with slices of tomato and lettuce, and assemble into sandwiches.

Ingredients: Chickpeas, lemon juice, Dijon mustard, fresh dill, celery, red onion, bell pepper, whole grain bread, lettuce, tomato.

Calories Count: Approximately 300-350 calories per serving.

Prep Time: 15 minutes.

Stuffed Bell Peppers with Quinoa and Black Beans:

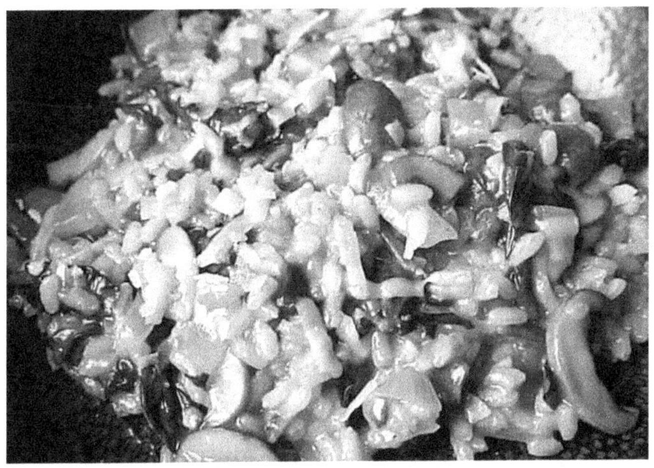

Stuffed bell peppers are a colorful and healthy option for a plant-based lunch. They are packed with quinoa, black beans, corn, and spices.

Method of Preparation:

Step 1: Cook quinoa per the directions on the package, then combine it with diced tomatoes, black beans, corn, cumin, and cilantro.

Step 2: After halving the bell peppers, stuff them with the mixture and bake them until they are soft. Serve hot with salsa and avocado slices.

Ingredients: Bell peppers, quinoa, black beans, corn, diced tomatoes, chili powder, cumin, cilantro, salsa, avocado.

Calories Count: Approximately 350-400 calories per serving.
Prep Time: 45 minutes.

Greek Salad with Tofu Feta:

This refreshing Greek salad will transport you to the Mediterranean with its flavors. It is topped with marinated tofu feta, crisp vegetables, olives, and a zesty vinaigrette.

Method of Preparation:

Step 1: Cube the tofu and let it marinate in garlic, olive oil, oregano, and lemon juice.

Step 2: Combine chopped romaine lettuce, cherry tomatoes, red onion, cucumber dice, and Kalamata olives.

Step 3: Tofu feta salad should be served with a balsamic vinaigrette drizzle.

Ingredients: Tofu, lemon juice, olive oil, oregano, garlic, cucumber, cherry tomatoes, red onion, Kalamata olives, romaine lettuce, balsamic vinaigrette.

Calories Count: Approximately 300-350 calories per serving.

Prep Time: 30 minutes.

Lentil and Vegetable Curry

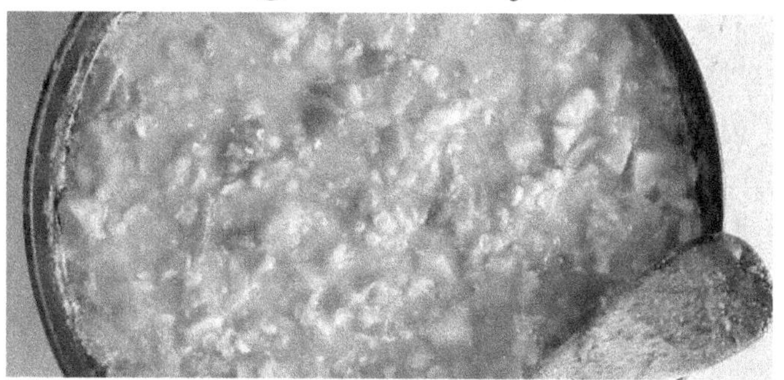

For a filling lunch option, warm up with a flavorful lentil and vegetable curry simmered in aromatic spices and coconut milk.

Method of Preparation:

Step 1: In a pot, sauté the ginger, garlic, and onions until fragrant.

Step 2: Add the cooked lentils, coconut milk, curry powder, turmeric, and chopped vegetables (carrots, potatoes, and cauliflower).

Step 3: Simmer until the curry thickens and the vegetables are soft. Over cooked brown rice, serve hot.

Ingredients: Lentils, onion, garlic, ginger, carrots, potatoes, cauliflower, curry powder, turmeric, coconut milk, brown rice.

Calories Count: Approximately 350-400 calories per serving.

Summer Harvest Salad with Balsamic Vinaigrette

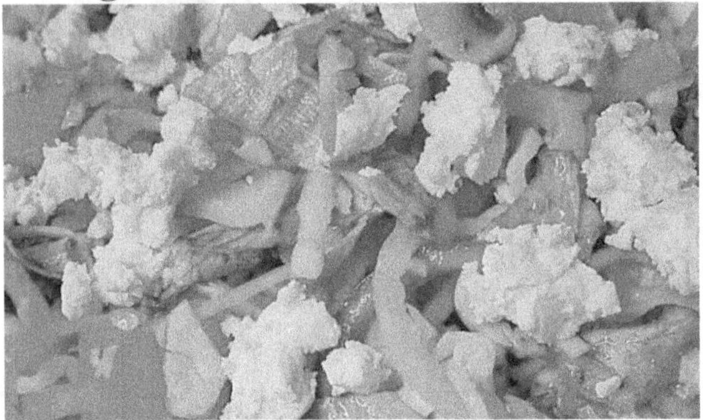

This colorful harvest salad, which features a variety of colorful fruits and vegetables tossed in a tart balsamic vinaigrette, is a great way to celebrate the flavors of summer.

Ingredients: Mixed greens, strawberries, blueberries, cherry tomatoes, cucumber, avocado, red onion, almonds, balsamic vinegar, olive oil, Dijon mustard, maple syrup, salt, pepper.

Preparation Method:
Step 1: Cucumber, strawberries, blueberries, cherry tomatoes, and mixed greens should all be cleaned and dried.

Step 2: Cut avocado, cucumber, and strawberries into slices. Slice red onion thinly and cut cherry tomatoes in half.

Step 3: In a dry skillet over medium heat, toast almonds until lightly golden, then coarsely chop.

Step 4: To make the dressing, combine the olive oil, maple syrup, Dijon mustard, balsamic vinegar, salt, and pepper in a small bowl.

Step 5: Combine sliced fruits and vegetables with mixed greens in a big bowl. Top with toasted almonds and a balsamic vinaigrette drizzle.

Calories Count: Approximately 250-300 calories per serving.

Prep Time: 15 minutes.

Mediterranean Quinoa Salad with Lemon-Herb Dressing:

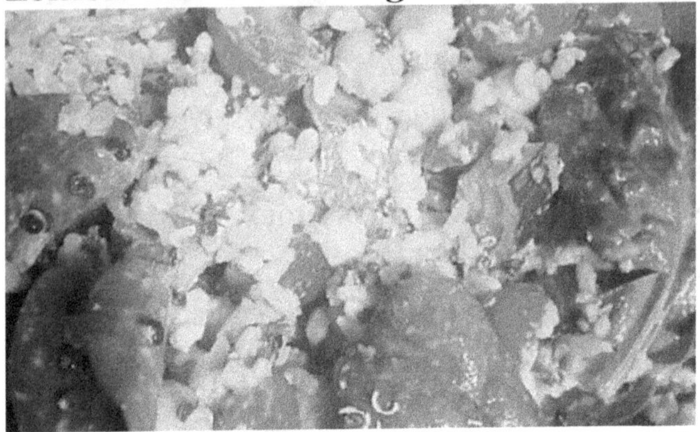

This vibrant quinoa salad will take your taste buds to the Mediterranean with its vibrant blend of veggies, olives, and herbs combined with a zesty lemon dressing.

Ingredients: Quinoa, cherry tomatoes, cucumber, bell peppers, Kalamata olives, red onion, parsley, lemon juice, olive oil, garlic, salt, pepper.

Preparation Method:

As directed on the package, prepare the quinoa and allow it to cool.

Step 1: Chop the red onion, bell peppers, cucumber, and cherry tomatoes. Cut parsley and remove pits from Kalamata olives.

Step 2: To make the dressing, combine the lemon juice, olive oil, minced garlic, salt, and pepper in a small bowl.

Step 3: Place cooked quinoa, chopped parsley, diced vegetables, and pitted Kalamata olives in a big bowl. Pour in the lemon-herb dressing and toss to ensure even coating.

Calories Count: Approximately 300-350 calories per serving.

Prep Time: 20 minutes.

Asian-Inspired Edamame and Mango Salad:

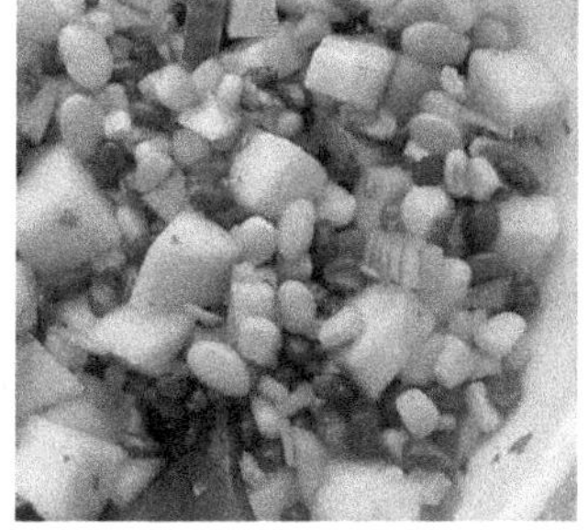

With sweet mango, crisp veggies, tangy sesame-ginger dressing, and protein-rich edamame, this Asian-inspired salad will tantalize your taste buds.

Ingredients: Edamame, mango, red cabbage, carrots, bell peppers, green onions, cilantro, sesame seeds, rice vinegar, soy sauce, sesame oil, ginger, garlic, maple syrup, lime juice.

Preparation Method: Cook edamame according to package instructions and let cool.

Step 1: Chop the mango, slice the bell peppers and green onions, julienne the carrots, shred the red cabbage. Toast the sesame seeds and chop the cilantro.

Step 2: To make dressing, combine rice vinegar, soy sauce, sesame oil, minced garlic and ginger, maple syrup, and lime juice in a small bowl.

Step 3: The cooked edamame, diced mango, shredded red cabbage, julienned carrots, sliced bell peppers, chopped cilantro, and sliced green onions should all be combined in a big bowl. **Step 4:** Sprinkle with toasted sesame seeds and drizzle with sesame-ginger dressing.

Calories Count: Approximately 300-350 calories per serving.

Prep Time: 25 minutes.

Roasted Beet and Walnut Salad with Creamy Cashew Dressing:

This dish of roasted beets, crunchy walnuts, and creamy cashew dressing will up your salad game and make for a filling and healthy supper.

Ingredients: Beets, mixed greens, walnuts, red onion, avocado, lemon juice, cashews, water, garlic, nutritional yeast, apple cider vinegar, Dijon mustard, salt, pepper.

Preparation Method:

Step 1: Preheat oven to 400°F (200°C). Individually wrap each beet in aluminum foil, then roast for 45 to 60 minutes, or until soft. Once cooled, peel and cut.

Step 2: Dice the avocado, thinly slice the red onion, and wash and dry the mixed greens. In a dry skillet over medium heat, toast walnuts until fragrant, then coarsely chop.

Step 3: To make the creamy cashew dressing, put the soaked cashews, water, nutritional yeast, minced garlic, apple cider vinegar, Dijon mustard, salt, and pepper in a blender.

Step 4: Combine diced avocado, toasted walnuts, thinly sliced red onion, and roasted beets with mixed greens in a big bowl. Serve with a drizzle of creamy cashew dressing.

Calories Count: Approximately 350-400 calories per serving.

Prep Time: 30 minutes.

Southwest Quinoa Salad with Avocado-Lime Dressing:

This quinoa salad with Southwest influences will liven up your usual salad rotation. It has creamy avocado-lime dressing, bell peppers, corn, and black beans for a taste explosion.

Ingredients: Quinoa, black beans, corn, avocado, lime juice, olive oil, cumin, chili powder, bell peppers, red onion, and cilantro.

Preparation Method:

Step 1: Cook quinoa according to package instructions and let cool.

Step 2: Drain and rinse the corn and black beans. Chop cilantro, slice red onion thinly, and dice bell peppers. To keep avocado from browning, chop it up and toss it with lime juice.

Step 3: To make the avocado-lime dressing, mash the avocado with the lime juice, olive oil, ground cumin, chili powder, salt, and pepper in a small bowl.

Step 4: Cooked quinoa, black beans, corn, diced bell peppers, thinly sliced red onion, and chopped cilantro should all be combined in a big bowl. Pour in the avocado-lime dressing and toss to ensure even coating.

Calories Count: Approximately 300-350 calories per serving.

Prep Time: 25 minutes.

Comforting Soups and Stews

Vegetable Lentil Soup:

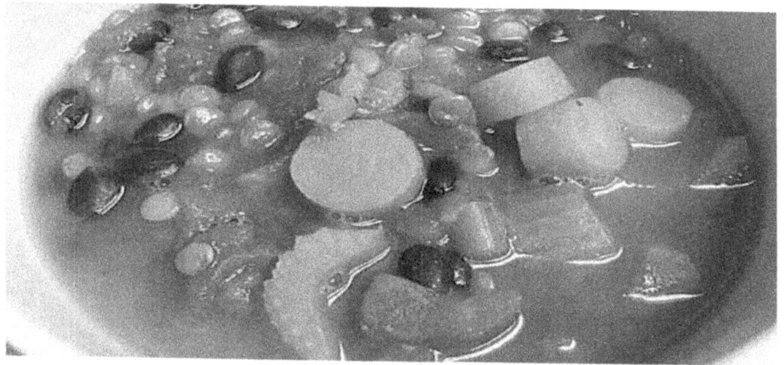

This filling and healthy vegetable lentil soup will help you warm up. It contains a lot of fiber-rich lentils, vibrant vegetables, and flavorful herbs and spices.

Ingredients: Lentils, vegetable broth, onion, carrots, celery, garlic, diced tomatoes, thyme, bay leaves, salt, pepper, parsley.

Preparation Method:

Step 1: Diced onion, carrots, and celery should be softened by sautéing them in olive oil in a big pot.

Step 2: Add the minced garlic and stir until fragrant, about 1 more minute.

Step 3: Lentils should be rinsed before being added to the pot with diced tomatoes, bay leaves, thyme, and vegetable broth.

Step 4: Once the soup is boiling, lower the heat and simmer it for twenty to twenty-five minutes, or until the lentils are soft.

Step 5: Serve hot, garnish with chopped parsley and season with salt and pepper to taste.

Calories Count: Approximately 200-250 calories per serving

Prep Time: 30 minutes.

Creamy Potato Leek Soup:

Savor the hearty flavors of this creamy potato leek soup, which is made with sautéed leeks, soft potatoes, and a hint of herbaceousness for a filling supper.

Ingredients: Potatoes, leeks, vegetable broth, garlic, thyme, nutmeg, salt, pepper, non-dairy milk (such as almond or soy), parsley.

Preparation Method:

Step 1: Dice and peel potatoes; slice only the white and light green portions of leeks.

Step 2: Sliced leeks should be softened by sautéing them in olive oil in a big pot.

Step 3: Saute the minced garlic for an additional minute, or until it becomes aromatic.

Step 4: Add nutmeg, thyme, and vegetable broth to the pot along with the diced potatoes.

Step 5: After bringing the soup to a boil, lower the heat, and simmer the potatoes for 20 to 25 minutes, or until they are tender.

Step 6: Blend the soup with an immersion blender until it is creamy and smooth.

Step 7: Serve hot, garnish with chopped parsley, season with salt and pepper to taste, and stir in non-dairy milk to desired consistency.

Calories Count: Approximately 250-300 calories per serving.

Prep Time: 35 minutes.

Are you enjoying this cookbook?

If you have any difficulty understanding the meals in this cookbook kindly reach out to me at mariakirby001@gmail.com.

For more awesome Cookbooks like this one make sure to scan this qr code.

Minestrone Soup:

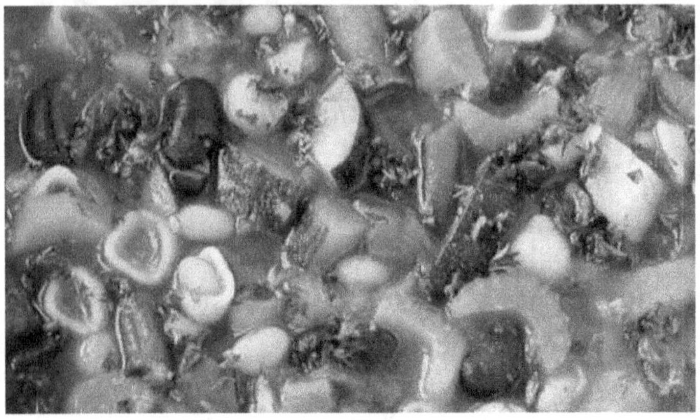

This comforting dish of hearty minestrone soup, loaded with beans, pasta, and Italian herbs, will let you savor the traditional flavors of Italy.

Ingredients: Vegetable broth, onion, garlic, carrots, celery, diced tomatoes, kidney beans, cannellini beans, small pasta (such as ditalini or elbow), spinach, Italian seasoning, salt, pepper, parsley, Parmesan cheese (optional).

Preparation Method:

Step 1: Diced onion, carrots, and celery should be softened by sautéing them in olive oil in a big pot.

Step 2: Once fragrant, add the minced garlic and cook for an additional minute.

Step 3: Drained and rinsed kidney and cannellini beans, diced tomatoes, vegetable broth, Italian seasoning, and pasta should all be added to the pot.

Step 4: Once the soup reaches a boil, lower the heat and simmer the pasta for ten to twelve minutes, or until it is al dente.

Step 5: Add the fresh spinach, stir, and cook until it wilts.

Step 6: Serve hot, garnish with grated Parmesan cheese and chopped parsley if desired, and season with salt and pepper to taste.

Calories Count: Approximately 250-300 calories per serving.

Prep Time: 40 minutes.

Curried Butternut Squash Soup:

This soup, which has the sweet flavors of butternut squash and aromatic spices, is creamy and aromatic, perfect for warming your soul.

Ingredients: Butternut squash, onion, garlic, vegetable broth, coconut milk, curry powder, ground cumin, ground coriander, ground ginger, salt, pepper, lime juice, cilantro.

Preparation Method:

Step 1: Chop the onion and garlic, and peel, seed, and dice the butternut squash.

Step 2: Add the chopped onion and garlic to a large pot and sauté in olive oil until softened.

Step 3: To the pot, add diced butternut squash, ground cumin, ground coriander, ground ginger, coconut milk, and vegetable broth.

Step 4: Once the squash is tender, simmer the soup for 20 to 25 minutes on low heat after bringing it to a boil.

Step 5: Blend the soup with an immersion blender until it is creamy and smooth.

Step 6: Serve hot, garnished with chopped cilantro and seasoned to taste with salt, pepper, and lime juice.

Calories Count: Approximately 200-250 calories per serving.

Prep Time: 35 minutes.

Hearty Vegetable Barley Stew:

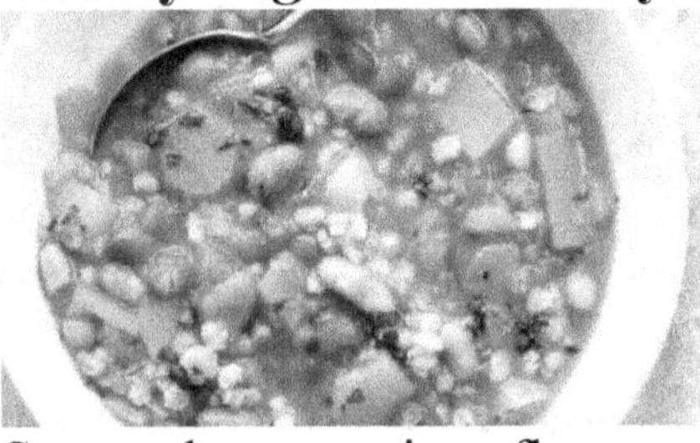

Savor the warming flavors of this filling and nutritious vegetable barley stew, which is made with tender barley, a variety of vegetables, and flavorful herbs.

Ingredients: Pearl barley, vegetable broth, onion, garlic, carrots, celery, potatoes, green beans, diced tomatoes, thyme, rosemary, salt, pepper, parsley.

Preparation Method:

Step 1: After rinsing in cold water, drain the pearl barley.

Step 2: Diced onion, carrots, and celery should be softened by sautéing them in olive oil in a big pot.

Step 3: Once fragrant, add the minced garlic and cook for an additional minute.

Step 4: To the pot, add the diced potatoes, cooked barley, diced tomatoes, green beans, vegetable broth, thyme, and rosemary.

Step 5: After bringing the stew to a boil, lower the heat, and simmer it for 25 to 30 minutes, or until the barley is cooked and the vegetables are soft.

Step 6: Serve hot, garnish with chopped parsley and season with salt and pepper to taste.

Calories Count: Approximately 250-300 calories per serving.

Prep Time: 45 minutes.

Tomato Basil Soup:

Savor the traditional pairing of juicy tomatoes and crisp basil in this warming tomato basil soup, ideal for a cosy midday meal.

Ingredients: Ripe tomatoes, onion, garlic, vegetable broth, fresh basil leaves, olive oil, salt, pepper, balsamic vinegar (optional), coconut cream (optional).

Preparation Method:

Step 1: Preheat oven to 400°F (200°C). Halve the tomatoes and arrange them cut-side up on a baking sheet. After sprinkling salt and pepper and drizzled with olive oil, roast the tomatoes for thirty to thirty-five minutes, or until they are soft and caramelized.

Step 2: Diced onion and minced garlic should be sautéed in olive oil in a big pot until they become soft.

Step 3: Toss in the roasted tomatoes with their juices, the vegetable broth, and the shredded basil leaves.

Step 4: Simmer the soup for fifteen to twenty minutes.

Step 5: Blend the soup with an immersion blender until it is smooth. Add a little bit of coconut cream or balsamic vinegar for extra flavor and creaminess, if preferred.

Step 7: Serve hot, garnished with fresh basil leaves and seasoned to taste with salt and pepper.

Calories Count: Approximately 150-200 calories per serving.

Prep Time: 50 minutes.

Chunky Vegetable Soup:

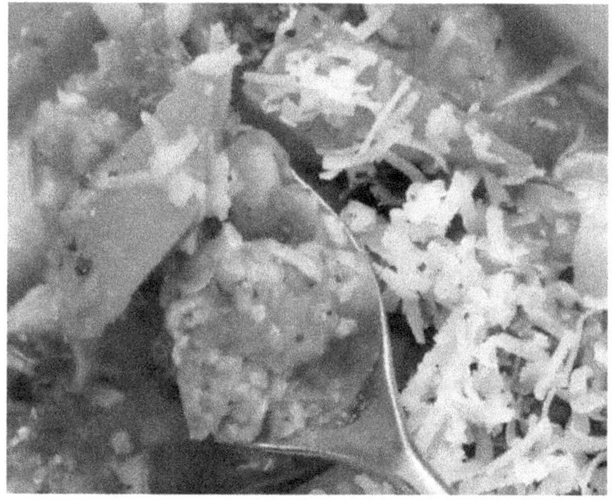

Enjoy a bowl of thick and filling chunky vegetable soup that is packed with a variety of vibrant veggies and flavorful herbs.

Ingredients: Vegetable broth, onion, garlic, carrots, celery, potatoes, green beans, corn kernels, diced tomatoes, thyme, rosemary, bay leaves, salt, pepper, parsley.

Preparation Method:

Step 1: Diced onion, carrots, and celery should be softened by sautéing them in olive oil in a big pot.

Step 2: Once fragrant, add the minced garlic and cook for an additional minute. To the pot, add the diced potatoes, green beans, corn kernels, diced tomatoes (with their juices), bay leaves, thyme, and rosemary.

Step 3: After bringing the soup to a boil, lower the heat, and simmer it until the vegetables are soft, 20 to 25 minutes.

Step 5: Serve hot, garnish with chopped parsley and season with salt and pepper to taste.

Calories Count: Approximately 200-250 calories per serving.

Prep Time: 40 minutes.

Coconut Curry Lentil Soup:

This coconut curry lentil soup, which has protein-rich lentils, spicy curry, and creamy coconut milk, will warm you up with its exotic flavors.

Ingredients: Red lentils, coconut milk, vegetable broth, onion, garlic, ginger, curry powder, ground turmeric, cayenne pepper, lime juice, cilantro.

Preparation Method:

Step 1: Drain and rinse red lentils under cold water.

Step 2: Add the minced garlic, grated ginger, and diced onion to a large pot and sauté in olive oil until softened.

Step 3: Cook for an additional minute or until fragrant after adding the cayenne pepper, curry powder, and ground turmeric to the pot.

Step 4: Pour the vegetable broth, coconut milk, and rinsed lentils into the pot. Once the soup has thickened and the lentils are cooked, bring it to a boil, then lower the heat and simmer for 20 to 25 minutes.

Step 5: Add the lime juice, taste and adjust the salt, add the chopped cilantro as a garnish, and serve hot.

Calories Count: Approximately 250-300 calories per serving.

Prep Time: 30 minutes.

Spicy Black Bean Soup:

This filling and savory spicy black bean soup will liven up your dinnertime. Packed with veggies, black beans, and a burst of chilli heat.

Ingredients: Black beans, vegetable broth, onion, garlic, bell pepper, diced tomatoes, chili powder, ground cumin, smoked paprika, cayenne pepper, lime juice, cilantro.

Preparation Method:

Step 1: Diced onion, minced garlic, and diced bell pepper should be softened by sautéing them in olive oil in a big pot.

Step 2: Pour in the diced tomatoes (with their juices), rinsed and drained black beans, vegetable broth, ground cumin, smoked paprika, chili powder, and cayenne.

Step 3: After bringing the soup to a boil, lower the heat, and simmer it for twenty to twenty-five minutes to let the flavors combine.

Step 4: Add the lime juice, taste and adjust the salt, add the chopped cilantro as a garnish, and serve hot.

Calories Count: Approximately 200-250 calories per serving.

Prep Time: 35 minutes.

Satisfying Dinners for Senior Satisfaction

Quinoa-Stuffed Bell Peppers:

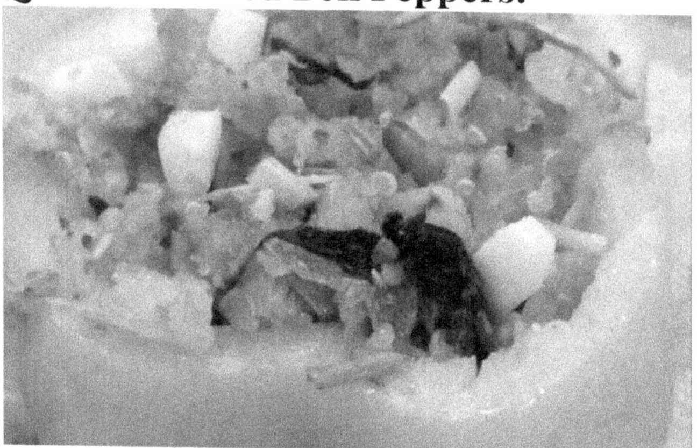

These vibrant bell peppers packed with a flavorful blend of quinoa, beans, veggies, and herbs will delight your palate.

Ingredients: Bell peppers, quinoa, vegetable broth, onion, garlic, black beans, corn kernels, diced tomatoes, cumin, paprika, chili powder, salt, pepper, cilantro.

Preparation Method:
1. Preheat the oven to 375°F (190°C). Slice off the bell peppers' tops, then take out the seeds and membranes.
2. Cook the quinoa in vegetable broth in a saucepan as directed on the package.

3. Diced onion and minced garlic should be cooked until transparent in a separate skillet.
4. To the skillet, add the cooked quinoa, diced tomatoes, black beans, and corn kernels. Cook until heated through.
5. Spoon the quinoa mixture into each bell pepper until filled to the top.
6. Place stuffed bell peppers in a baking dish and bake for 25-30 minutes, or until peppers are tender.
7. Garnish with fresh cilantro before serving.

Calories Count: Approximately 300-350 calories per serving.
Prep Time: 45 minutes.

Chickpea and Vegetable Stir-Fry:

Enjoy a quick and flavorful dinner with this chickpea and vegetable stir-fry, featuring a colorful array of vegetables and protein-rich chickpeas in a savory sauce.

Ingredients: Chickpeas, bell peppers, broccoli, carrots, snap peas, onion, garlic, ginger, soy sauce, sesame oil, rice vinegar, maple syrup, cornstarch, green onions, sesame seeds.

Preparation Method:

1. Drain and rinse chickpeas and pat dry with a paper towel.
2. In a wok or large skillet, heat sesame oil over medium heat. Add minced garlic and grated ginger, and sauté until fragrant.
3. Add sliced onion, bell peppers, broccoli florets, sliced carrots, and snap peas to the skillet. Stir-fry until vegetables are tender-crisp.
4. In a small bowl, whisk together soy sauce, rice vinegar, maple syrup, and cornstarch to make the sauce.
5. Add drained chickpeas and sauce to the skillet, stirring until everything is well coated and heated through.
6. Serve hot, garnished with sliced green onions and sesame seeds.

Calories Count: Approximately 250-300 calories per serving.

Prep Time: 30 minutes.

Eggplant Parmesan:

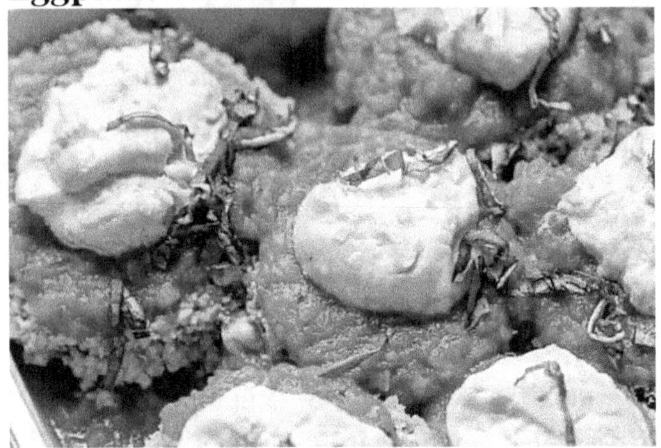

Indulge in a classic Italian favorite with this plant-based eggplant Parmesan, featuring crispy breaded eggplant slices topped with marinara sauce and vegan cheese.

Ingredients: Eggplant, breadcrumbs, nutritional yeast, Italian seasoning, marinara sauce, vegan mozzarella cheese, fresh basil.

Preparation Method:

1. Preheat the oven to 400°F (200°C). Slice the eggplant into 1/2-inch rounds.

2. In a shallow dish, mix breadcrumbs, nutritional yeast, and Italian seasoning. Dip eggplant slices into the breadcrumb mixture, coating both sides evenly.

3. Place breaded eggplant slices on a baking sheet lined with parchment paper. Bake for

20-25 minutes, flipping halfway through, until golden brown and crispy.

4. Remove the baking sheet from the oven. Spoon marinara sauce over each eggplant slice and sprinkle with vegan mozzarella cheese.
5. Return the baking sheet to the oven and bake for an additional 10-15 minutes, or until the cheese is melted and bubbly.
6. Garnish with fresh basil before serving.

Calories Count: Approximately 300-350 calories per serving.
Prep Time: 45 minutes.

Lentil Shepherd's Pie:

Dive into comfort with this hearty lentil shepherd's pie, featuring a savory lentil and vegetable filling topped with creamy mashed potatoes.

Ingredients: Brown lentils, potatoes, vegetable broth, onion, carrots, peas, garlic, tomato paste, thyme, rosemary, olive oil, non-dairy milk, nutritional yeast, salt, pepper.

Preparation Method:

1. Preheat the oven to 400°F (200°C). Peel and dice potatoes, then boil in a pot of salted

water until tender. Drain and mash with non-dairy milk, nutritional yeast, salt, and pepper.
2. In a separate pot, cook brown lentils in vegetable broth until tender.
3. In a skillet, sauté diced onion, minced garlic, sliced carrots, and peas until softened. Add cooked lentils, tomato paste, thyme, and rosemary to the skillet, stirring to combine.
4. Transfer the lentil and vegetable mixture to a baking dish. Spread mashed potatoes evenly over the top.
5. Bake for 25-30 minutes, or until the mashed potatoes are lightly golden.
6. Let cool for a few minutes before serving.

Calories Count: Approximately 300-350 calories per serving.
Prep Time: 60 minutes.

Chickpea and Spinach Coconut Curry:

Enjoy a taste of India with this aromatic chickpea and spinach coconut curry, featuring creamy coconut milk, tender chickpeas, and flavorful spices.
Ingredients: Chickpeas, spinach, onion, garlic, ginger, curry powder, ground turmeric, cumin, coconut milk, diced tomatoes, vegetable broth, lime juice, cilantro.

Preparation Method:

1. In a large skillet, sauté diced onion, minced garlic, and grated ginger in olive oil until softened.
2. Add curry powder, ground turmeric, and ground cumin to the skillet, stirring until fragrant.
3. Stir in diced tomatoes (with juices), coconut milk, and vegetable broth. Bring to a simmer.
4. Add drained chickpeas and chopped spinach to the skillet, cooking until spinach is wilted and chickpeas are heated through.
5. Stir in lime juice and season with salt and pepper to taste.
6. Garnish with chopped cilantro before serving.

Calories Count: Approximately 250-300 calories per serving.

Prep Time: 30 minutes.

Mushroom and Spinach Risotto:

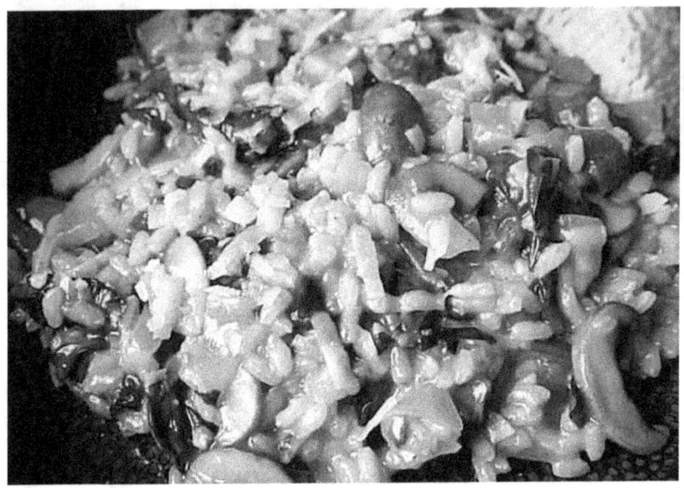

Indulge in creamy comfort with this mushroom and spinach risotto, featuring Arborio rice cooked to perfection in a flavorful mushroom broth.

Ingredients: Arborio rice, mushrooms, vegetable broth, onion, garlic, white wine (optional), nutritional yeast, spinach, thyme, olive oil, salt, pepper, parsley.

Preparation Method:

1. In a saucepan, heat vegetable broth and keep it warm over low heat.
2. In a separate skillet, sauté diced onion and minced garlic in olive oil until translucent. Add sliced mushrooms to the skillet and cook until browned and tender.

3. Add Arborio rice to the skillet and stir to coat in the oil.
4. Deglaze the skillet with white wine (if using) and cook until the liquid has evaporated.
5. Begin adding warm vegetable broth to the skillet, one ladleful at a time, stirring constantly and allowing the rice to absorb the liquid before adding more.
6. Continue this process until the rice is creamy and tender, about 20-25 minutes.
7. Stir in nutritional yeast, chopped spinach, and fresh thyme.
8. Season with salt and pepper to taste, garnish with chopped parsley, and serve hot.

Calories Count: Approximately 300-350 calories per serving.

Prep Time: 45 minutes.

Stuffed Portobello Mushrooms:

Elevate your dinner with these flavorful stuffed portobello mushrooms, filled with a savory mixture of quinoa, vegetables, and herbs, topped with melted vegan cheese.

Ingredients: Portobello mushrooms, quinoa, vegetable broth, onion, garlic, bell pepper, spinach, cherry tomatoes, balsamic vinegar, Italian seasoning, vegan mozzarella cheese, basil.

Preparation Method:

1. Preheat the oven to 375°F (190°C). Remove the stems and gills from the portobello mushrooms and place them on a baking sheet.
2. Cook quinoa in vegetable broth according to package instructions.
3. In a skillet, sauté diced onion and minced garlic until translucent. Add diced bell pepper, chopped spinach, halved cherry tomatoes, cooked quinoa, balsamic vinegar, and Italian seasoning. Cook until vegetables are tender.
4. Spoon the quinoa mixture into each portobello mushroom cap, pressing down gently.
5. Top each mushroom with vegan mozzarella cheese.
6. Bake for 20-25 minutes, or until mushrooms are tender and cheese is melted.
7. Garnish with fresh basil before serving.

Calories Count: Approximately 250-300 calories per serving.

Prep Time: 40 minutes.

Walnut Pesto Pasta Salad

A light and cool pasta salad that is ideal for a warm day. The walnuts are a great source of omega-3 fatty acids and add a nice crunch.

Ingredients: Whole wheat pasta, Fresh basil leaves, Walnuts, Garlic cloves, Olive oil, Cherry tomatoes, Roasted red peppers, Salt and pepper to taste

Preparation Instructions

1. Prepare the pasta per the directions on the package, then set aside to cool.
2. To make the pesto, pulse the basil, walnuts, garlic, and olive oil in a food processor.
3. Mix the pesto into the pasta.
4. Include the roasted red peppers and cherry tomatoes.
5. Add pepper and salt for seasoning.

Calories: Approximately 450 calories per serving.
Prep Time: 20 minutes.

Tofu Tacos

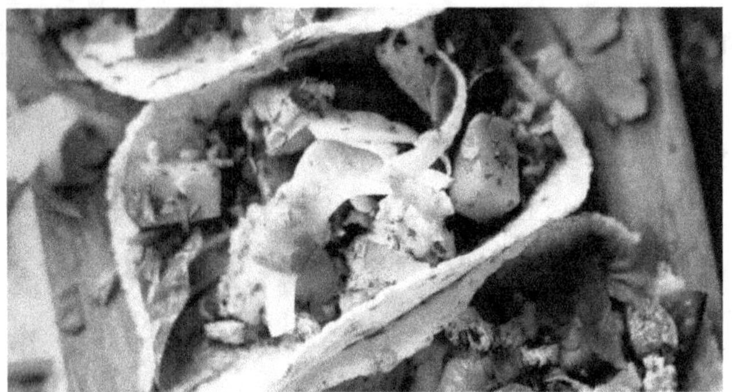

A spicy tofu mixture fills these tacos, adding a zesty flavor to your mealtime.

Ingredients

- Firm tofu
- Taco seasoning
- Olive oil
- Corn tortillas
- Shredded cabbage
- Pico de gallo
- Guacamole

Preparation Instructions

1. Crumble the tofu and sauté with taco seasoning and olive oil until browned.
2. Warm the tortillas in a pan.
3. Fill tortillas with the tofu mixture.
4. Top with shredded cabbage, pico de gallo, and guacamole.

Calories: Approximately 300 calories per serving.
Prep Time: 15 minutes.

Spinach & Mushroom Quiche

A crustless quiche that's simple to make and filled with the goodness of spinach and mushrooms.

Ingredients:
- Fresh spinach
- Sliced mushrooms
- Eggs
- Grated Gruyère cheese
- Milk
- Nutmeg
- Salt and pepper

Preparation Instructions
1. Preheat the oven to 375°F (190°C).
2. Add the spinach and sauté until it wilts.
3. Beat eggs, cheese, milk, nutmeg, pepper, and salt together.
4. Include the sautéed veggies in the mixture of eggs.
5. Transfer to an oiled pie plate and bake for thirty-five minutes.

Calories: Approximately 200 calories per slice.
Prep Time: 45 minutes.

Vegan Mushroom Bolognese

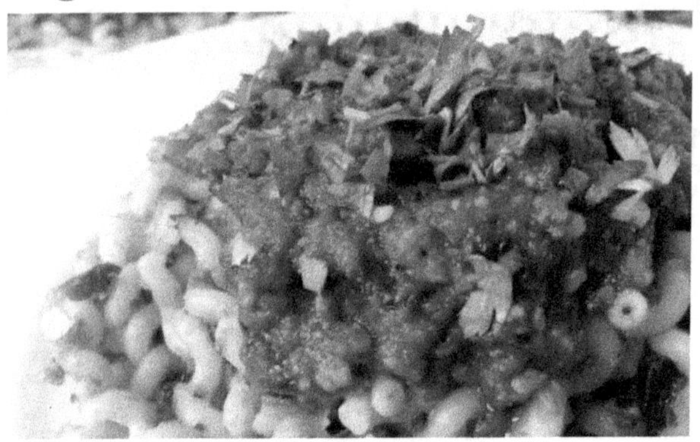

A filling bolognese sauce with a mushroom base that is perfect for a hefty supper.

Ingredients:
- Button mushrooms
- Onion
- Garlic
- Carrots
- Celery
- Canned tomatoes
- White wine
- Olive oil
- Salt and pepper
- Whole wheat spaghetti

Preparation Instructions
1. Chop the celery, carrots, onion, and garlic finely.
2. Sauté in a little olive oil until tender.

3. Simmer for 30 minutes after adding canned tomatoes and white wine.
4. Add pepper and salt for seasoning.
5. Top with cooked spaghetti made with whole wheat.

Calories: Approximately 350 calories per serving.
Prep Time: 1 hour.

Arepas with Spicy Black Beans

A traditional Latin American dish, arepas are corn cakes that can be split and filled with a variety of toppings.

Ingredients:

- Precooked cornmeal
- Warm water
- Salt
- Cooked black beans
- Spices (cumin, paprika, chili powder)
- Avocado
- Fresh cilantro

Preparation Instructions

1. To make a dough, combine cornmeal, warm water, and salt.
2. Form into patties and sear until golden on a hot griddle.
3. Combine spices with black beans and cook.
4. Divide arepas and stuff with hot black beans.

5. Add sliced avocado and cilantro on top.

Calories: Approximately 400 calories per serving.
Prep Time: 30 minutes.

Nutrient-Dense Side Dishes

Roasted Brussels Sprouts with Balsamic Glaze

Perfectly caramelized, these roasted Brussels sprouts are topped with a tart and sweet balsamic glaze.

Ingredients:

- 1 lb Brussels sprouts, halved
- Two tablespoons of olive oil
- Salt and pepper to taste
– 2 tablespoons balsamic vinegar
- One teaspoon of maple syrup

Preparation Instructions:

1. Preheat your oven to 400°F (200°C).
2. Add salt, pepper, and olive oil to the Brussels sprouts and toss.
3. After spreading them out on a baking sheet, roast them for 20 to 25 minutes, or until crispy.
4. Combine maple syrup and balsamic vinegar in a whisk.

5. Before serving, drizzle the glaze over the roasted Brussels sprouts.

Calories: Approximately 100 calories per serving.
Prep Time: 30 minutes.

Quinoa Tabbouleh

Usually made with bulgur, tabbouleh is a light and refreshing Middle Eastern salad. Here, however, it is made with quinoa, which is high in protein.

Ingredients:
One cup of cooked quinoa.
- One cup of finely chopped parsley
- 1/4 cup finely chopped mint
- Two diced tomatoes
- One diced cucumber
- One diced cucumber
- Two tablespoons of olive oil
- Salt to taste

Preparation Instructions
1. In a bowl, mix cooked quinoa, cucumber, tomatoes, parsley, and mint.
2. Combine salt, olive oil, and lemon juice in a different bowl.
3. Drizzle the quinoa mixture with the dressing and mix thoroughly.
4. Before serving, let it cool in the fridge.

Calories: Approximately 150 calories per serving.

Prep Time: 20 minutes.

Sweet Potato and Kale Hash

A delicious and nutritious hash that is hearty and colorful.

Ingredients:

- Two diced sweet potatoes
- One bunch of chopped kale leaves, with the stems removed
- One chopped onion
- Two tablespoons of olive oil

To taste, add salt and pepper.

Preparation Instructions:

1. In a big skillet over medium heat, warm up the olive oil.
2. Add the chopped onions and sweet potatoes, and cook until soft.
3. Add the kale and toss, cooking until it wilts.
4. To taste, add salt and pepper for seasoning.

Calories: Approximately 200 calories per serving.

Prep Time: 25 minutes.

Steamed Green Beans with Almond Slivers

Crunchy almonds combined with crisp green beans create a straightforward but sophisticated side dish.

Ingredients:

- 1 lb green beans, trimmed
- 1/4 cup almond slivers
- 1 tbsp olive oil
- Salt to taste

Preparation Instructions

1. Steamed green beans should be crisp-tender.
2. Toast almond slivers in a pan until it becomes golden brown.
3. Combine toasted almonds and olive oil with the steamed green beans.
4. Add salt to the food before serving.

Calories: Approximately 80 calories per serving.
Prep Time: 15 minutes.

Moroccan Carrot Salad

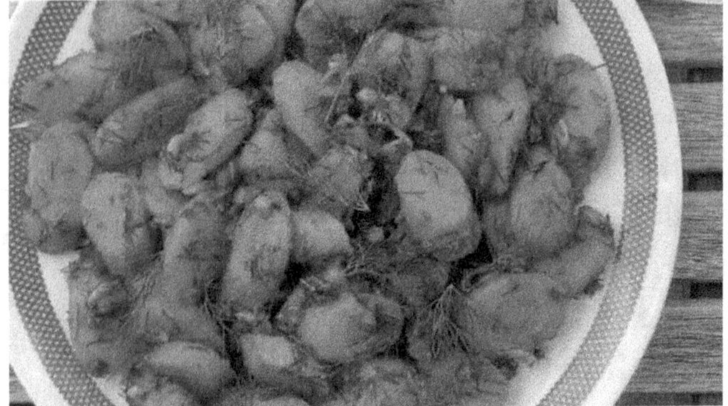

This salad adds color and vibrancy to any meal because it is loaded with flavors from the herbs and spices.

Ingredients:

- 4 large carrots, grated
- 1/4 cup raisins
- 2 tbsp lemon juice
- 2 tbsp olive oil
- 1 tsp cumin
- 1/2 tsp cinnamon
- 1/4 cup fresh cilantro, chopped
- Salt to taste

Preparation Instructions:

1. Combine the raisins and grated carrots in a big bowl.
2. Combine the lemon juice, cinnamon, cumin, and olive oil in a small bowl.

3. Drizzle the carrot mixture with the dressing, then thoroughly toss.
4. Add the chopped cilantro and sprinkle some salt on top.

Calories: Approximately 120 calories per serving.
Prep Time: 15 minutes.

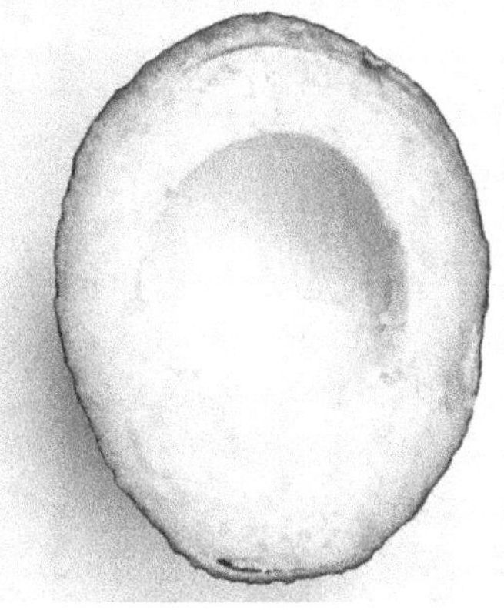

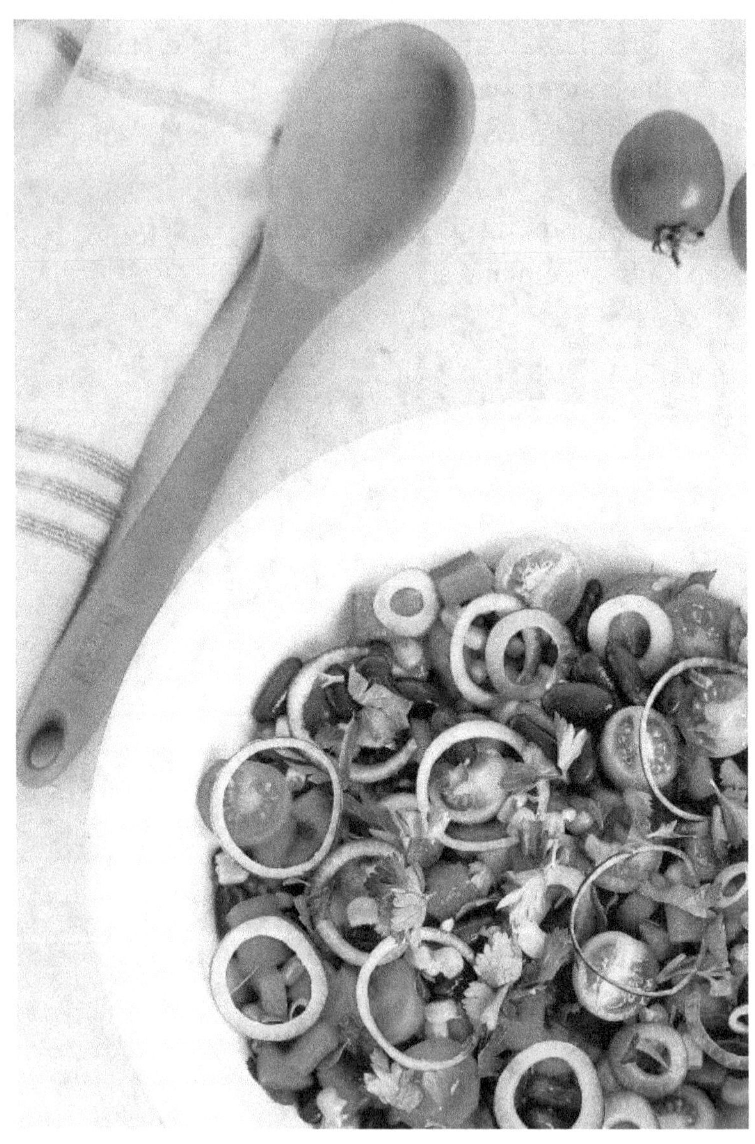

Healthy Dessert Options for Occasional Indulgence

Chia Seed Pudding with Mixed Berries

Rich in omega-3 fatty acids and fiber, chia seed pudding is a tasty and healthful dessert. It is a satisfying and healthful sweet treat that is topped with fresh mixed berries.

Ingredients:

- 1/4 cup chia seeds
- 1 cup unsweetened almond milk
- 1 tbsp maple syrup
- 1/2 tsp vanilla extract
- Mixed berries (strawberries, blueberries, raspberries)

Preparation Instructions

1. Combine the almond milk, vanilla extract, maple syrup, and chia seeds in a bowl.
2. Once it reaches the consistency of pudding, cover and chill for at least two hours.
3. Garnish with an abundance of mixed berries.

Calories: Approximately 150 calories per serving.

Prep Time: 2 hours 10 minutes.

Baked Cinnamon Apples

Easy to prepare and naturally sweet, baked cinnamon apples make a warm and comforting dessert.

Ingredients:

- 4 large apples, cored and sliced
- 2 tsp ground cinnamon
- 1/4 cup raisins
- 1/4 cup chopped walnuts
- 1/4 cup water

Preparation Instructions

1. Preheat the oven to 350°F (175°C).
2. Put the apple slices in a baking dish with cinnamon on top.
3. Scatter raisins and walnuts over the apples.
4. Add water to the dish and bake until the apples are tender, about 30 minutes.

Calories: Approximately 120 calories per serving.
Prep Time: 40 minutes.

Avocado Chocolate Mousse

Avocado serves as the foundation for this rich chocolate mousse, giving it a smooth texture and a heart-healthy fat source.

Ingredients:

- 2 ripe avocados

- 1/4 cup cocoa powder
- 1/4 cup almond milk
- 2 tbsp maple syrup
- 1 tsp vanilla extract

Preparation Instructions:

1. Scoop out the flesh from the avocado and transfer it to a blender.
2. Include vanilla extract, almond milk, maple syrup, and cocoa powder.
3. Blend until creamy and smooth.
4. Before serving, let it cool in the fridge.

Calories: Approximately 200 calories per serving.

Prep Time: 1 hour 10 minutes.

Coconut Yogurt Parfait

A parfait is a dessert in layers that frequently consists of granola, fruit, and yogurt. To make this version dairy-free, coconut yogurt is used instead.

Ingredients:

- 1 cup coconut yogurt
- 1/2 cup granola
- 1/2 cup fresh fruit (kiwi, mango, or berries)
- A drizzle of honey (optional)

Preparation Instructions:

1. Spoon a layer of coconut yogurt into a glass.
2. Add a layer of granola.
3. Add a layer of fresh fruit.

4. Repeat the layers until the glass is full.
5. Drizzle with honey if desired.
Calories: Approximately 250 calories per serving.
Prep Time: 10 minutes.

Peanut Butter Banana Ice Cream

This ice cream alternative is made with frozen bananas and peanut butter, creating a creamy and delicious treat.

Ingredients:
- 3 ripe bananas, sliced and frozen
- 2 tbsp peanut butter
- 1/4 tsp cinnamon

Preparation Instructions:
1. Place frozen banana slices in a food processor.
2. Add peanut butter and cinnamon.
3. Process the mixture until it has the consistency and smoothness of soft-serve ice cream.
4. For a firmer texture, serve right away or freeze.
Calories: Approximately 180 calories per serving.
Prep Time: 10 minutes (plus freezing time for bananas).

Snack Ideas for Boosting Energy and Satiety

Almond Butter Stuffed Dates

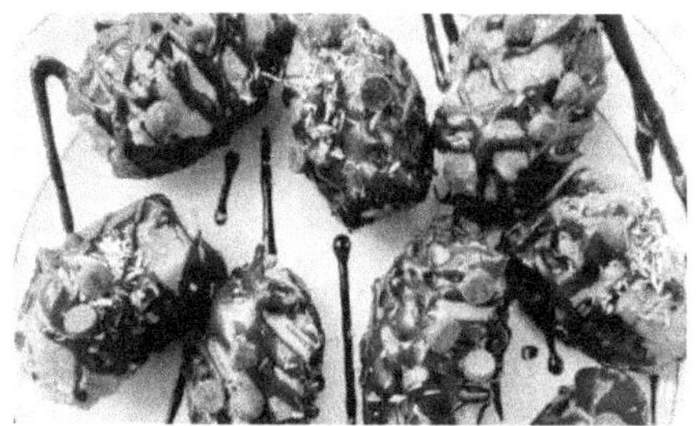

Almond butter-filled dates are a delightful and filling snack that offer a healthy ratio of natural sugars and fats.

Ingredients:

- Medjool dates
- Almond butter

Preparation Instructions:

1. If the dates have not been pitted already, pit them.
2. Place a teaspoon of almond butter inside each date.

Calories: Approximately 100 calories per serving (2 stuffed dates).

Prep Time: 5 minutes.

Veggie Sticks with Beet Hummus

A colorful and visually appealing snack that is high in nutrients is crunchy vegetable sticks dipped in vibrant beet hummus.

Ingredients:

- Assorted vegetables (carrots, celery, bell peppers)
- Cooked beets
- Chickpeas
- Tahini
- Lemon juice
- Garlic
- Olive oil
- Salt

Preparation Instructions:

1. In a food processor, blend together cooked beets, chickpeas, tahini, lemon juice, garlic, and olive oil until smooth.
2. Add salt to taste as a seasoning.
3. Chop veggies into sticks so you can dip them.

Calories: Approximately 150 calories per serving.
Prep Time: 15 minutes.

Spiced Pumpkin Seeds

Pumpkin seeds are a fantastic way to get zinc and magnesium. Roasting them with spices turns them into a tasty and crunchy snack.

Ingredients:

- Pumpkin seeds
- Olive oil
- Paprika
- Garlic powder
- Salt

Preparation Instructions:

1. Preheat the oven to 350°F (175°C).
2. Combine salt, paprika, garlic powder, and a small amount of olive oil with pumpkin seeds.
3. Spread out onto a baking sheet, then roast until crispy, 10 to 15 minutes.

Calories: Approximately 180 calories per serving (1/4 cup).

Prep Time: 20 minutes.

Avocado Rice Cakes

A heart-healthy, low-complication snack that is high in fiber and monounsaturated fats is avocado spread on rice cakes.

Ingredients:

- Rice cakes
- Ripe avocado
- Lemon juice
- Salt and pepper

Preparation Instructions:
1. Mash the avocado with salt, pepper, and lemon juice.
2. Spread the mixture on rice cakes.

Calories: Approximately 120 calories per serving (1 rice cake with avocado).

Prep Time: 5 minute

Oatmeal Energy Balls

Fiber and protein-rich oatmeal energy balls are a portable and practical snack that will keep you feeling full and energized.

Ingredients:
- Rolled oats
- Peanut butter
- Honey or maple syrup
- Chia seeds
- Dried cranberries or raisins

Preparation Instructions:
1. In a bowl, combine rolled oats, peanut butter, chia seeds, honey or maple syrup, and dried cranberries.
2. Form the mixture into tiny balls.

3. To set, chill in the refrigerator.

Calories: Approximately 90 calories per ball.

Prep Time: 15 minutes (plus chilling time).

Sweet and Savory Treats for Special Occasions

Avocado Chocolate Mousse

A creamy and rich dessert that's both indulgent and healthy.

Ingredients:

2 ripe avocados

1/4 cup cocoa powder

1/4 cup almond milk

1/3 cup maple syrup

1 teaspoon vanilla extract

Pinch of salt

Preparation Instructions:

1. Remove the avocado flesh with a spoon and transfer it to a blender.

2. Mix in the almond milk, vanilla extract, maple syrup, cocoa powder, and a small amount of salt.

3. Blend until creamy and smooth.

4. Before serving, let the food cool for at least an hour in the refrigerator.

Calories: Approximately 200 per serving.
Prep Time: 10 minutes + chilling time.

Stuffed Bell Peppers

Vibrant bell peppers packed with a tasty blend of quinoa and vegetables.

Ingredients:

4 large bell peppers, any color

1 cup cooked quinoa

1/2 cup black beans, drained and rinsed

1/2 cup corn kernels

1/2 cup diced tomatoes

1 teaspoon cumin

1 teaspoon paprika

Salt and pepper to taste

Preparation Instructions:

1. Preheat the oven to 350°F (175°C).
2. Slice off the bell peppers' tops, then take out the seeds.
3. Quinoa, black beans, corn, diced tomatoes, cumin, paprika, salt, and pepper should all be combined in a bowl.
4. After stuffing the bell peppers with the mixture, put them in a baking dish.
5. Bake the peppers for 25 to 30 minutes, or until they are soft.

Calories: Approximately 150 per stuffed pepper.
Prep Time: 15 minutes + baking time.

Carrot and Walnut Cake

A cake that is flavorful and moist, ideal for a celebration.

Ingredients:

2 cups grated carrots

1 cup whole wheat flour

1/2 cup chopped walnuts

1/2 cup apple sauce

1/4 cup almond milk

1/4 cup maple syrup

1 teaspoon baking soda

1 teaspoon cinnamon

1/2 teaspoon nutmeg

Preparation Instructions:

1. Preheat the oven to 350°F (175°C).
2. Grated carrots, flour, walnuts, apple sauce, almond milk, maple syrup, baking soda, cinnamon, and nutmeg should all be combined in a big bowl.
3. Fill a cake pan with oil and pour the batter into it.
4. A toothpick inserted into the center should come out clean after baking for 30 to 35 minutes.

Calories: Approximately 250 per slice.
Prep Time: 20 minutes + baking time.

Savory Mushroom Tartlets

Tartlets are a classy and savory appetizer.
Ingredients:
1 sheet of vegan puff pastry
1 cup sliced mushrooms
1/2 cup chopped onions
1 tablespoon olive oil
1 teaspoon thyme
Salt and pepper to taste
Preparation Instructions:
1. Preheat the oven to 400°F (200°C).
2. In a pan, heat olive oil and sauté onions and mushrooms with thyme, salt, and pepper until tender.
3. Cut the puff pastry into small squares and press into mini muffin tins.
4. Spoon the mushroom mixture into the pastry cups.
5. Bake for 12-15 minutes until the pastry is golden brown.

Calories: Approximately 100 per tartlet.
Prep Time: 20 minutes + baking time.

Sweet Potato and Black Bean Empanadas

A delicious and filling dessert with a hint of Latin America.

Ingredients:

2 cups mashed sweet potatoes

1 cup black beans, drained and rinsed

1 teaspoon cumin

1/2 teaspoon chili powder

1 sheet of vegan pie crust

Preparation Instructions:

1. Preheat the oven to 375°F (190°C).
2. Combine black beans, cumin, chili powder, and mashed sweet potatoes in a bowl.
3. Pie crust should be rolled out and cut into circles.
4. Spoon a portion of the sweet potato mixture onto each circle's half.
5. Using a fork, fold over and seal the edges.
6. Bake the crust for 20 to 25 minutes, or until golden brown.

Calories: Approximately 200 per empanada.

Prep Time: 30 minutes + baking time.

Hydrating Beverage Options

Cucumber Mint Water

A cool, hydrating beverage that is ideal on hot days.

Ingredients:

1 large cucumber, thinly sliced
10 fresh mint leaves
2 liters of water
Preparation:
1. Add the mint leaves and cucumber slices to a large pitcher.
2. Pour water into the pitcher and give it a gentle stir.
3. Let the flavors steep for at least an hour by placing it in the refrigerator.
4. Serve chilled.

Calories: Less than 10 per glass.
Prep Time: 5 minutes + infusion time.

Lemon Ginger Tea

A warming, calming drink that is good for the digestive system.

Ingredients:
1-inch piece of ginger, peeled and sliced
1/2 lemon, juiced
1 teaspoon honey (optional, for sweetness)
1 cup of hot water

Preparation Instructions:
1. Put the slices of ginger in a mug.
2. After covering the ginger with hot water, let it steep for five minutes.
3. Remove the ginger pieces from the water by straining.
4. If desired, stir in the honey and lemon juice.
5. Serve warm.

Calories: Approximately 25 per cup (with honey).
Prep Time: 10 minutes.

Watermelon Basil Cooler

A flavorful, hydrating beverage with a sweet, aromatic taste.

Ingredients:

2 cups cubed watermelon

5-6 basil leaves

1 cup coconut water

Ice cubes

Preparation Instructions:

1. Blend the watermelon cubes and basil leaves until smooth.
2. Strain the mixture to remove any pulp.
3. Mix the strained juice with coconut water.
4. Serve over ice cubes.

Calories: About 50 per serving.
Prep Time: 10 minutes.

Peach Iced Tea

A fruity twist on traditional iced tea, naturally sweetened with ripe peaches.

Ingredients:

2 ripe peaches, pitted and sliced

4 cups of water

2 tea bags (green or black tea)

Ice cubes

Preparation Instructions:

1. In a saucepan, bring water to a boil and add the tea bags.
2. Lower the heat and simmer for 5 minutes.
3. Remove the tea bags and let the tea cool.
4. In a blender, puree the peach slices.
5. Mix the peach puree with the cooled tea.
6. Serve over ice cubes.

Calories: Approximately 30 per glass.
Prep Time: 15 minutes + cooling time.

Carrot Orange Juice

A vitamin-packed juice with orange zest and carrot sweetness combined.

Ingredients:

5 large carrots, peeled
2 oranges, peeled and seeds removed
1-inch piece of turmeric root (optional)

Preparation:
1. Use a juicer to juice the oranges, carrots, and turmeric root.
2. To mix the flavors, stir the juice.
3. Either serve right away or refrigerate.

Calories: Around 120 per serving.
Prep Time: 10 minutes.

These drinks are perfect for you to enjoy on any occasion because they are not only delicious but also hydration-rich and nutrient-dense.

Importance of Social Connection and Community

The value of community and social interaction becomes more and more apparent as you age. Developing deep connections with people and interacting with them can have a significant positive impact on your general wellbeing. Developing a feeling of support and community within your community is crucial.

You can create new friendships and deepen current ones by taking part in social events, clubs, or volunteer work. The company, emotional support, and sense of purpose that these relationships offer are essential for preserving mental and emotional well-being.

Becoming a part of a community also presents chances for growth, learning, and shared experiences. Surrounded by people who share your interests, whether it is through local events, hobby clubs, or religious or cultural gatherings, can make your life happier and more fulfilling.

Furthermore, having a support system in place can help when needed, whether it is just someone to talk to or assistance with everyday chores or emotional support during trying times.

In the end, making social interaction a priority and getting involved in your community can result in a richer and more satisfying life as you age. Recognize that you are a vital part of something bigger than yourself and seize the chance to interact with people and give back to your community.

14 DAYS MEAL PLAN

Breakfast:	Lunch:	Dinner:	Desserts:
Day 1			
Berry Oatmeal Smoothie Bowl	Chickpea and Vegetable Stir-Fry	Walnut Pesto Pasta Salad	Avocado Chocolate Mousse
Day 2			
Mango Coconut Chia Pudding	Lentil Soup with Spinach and Lemon	Tofu Tacos	Baked Cinnamon Apples
Day 3			
Pineapple Ginger Green Smoothie	Mediterranean Stuffed Portobello Mushrooms	Vegan Mushroom Bolognese	Coconut Yogurt Parfait
Day 4			

Apple Cinnamon Baked Oatmeal	Quinoa Tabbouleh Salad	Arepas with Spicy Black Beans	Chia Seed Pudding with Mixed Berries
Day 5			
Hummus and Veggie Wrap	Spinach & Mushroom Quiche	Chickpea and Spinach Coconut Curry	Peanut Butter Banana Ice Cream
Day 6			
Quinoa Tabbouleh	Lentil Shepherd's Pie	Mushroom and Spinach Risotto	Avocado Rice Cakes
Day 7			
Banana Walnut Breakfast Cookies	Moroccan Chickpea Stew	Roasted Brussels Sprouts with Balsamic Glaze	Oatmeal Energy Balls

Day 8			
Chickpea and Spinach Coconut Curry	Vegan Mushroom Bolognese	Falafel Pita Sandwich with Tzatziki Sauce	Baked Cinnam on Apples
Day 9			
Berry Oatmeal Smoothie Bowl	Minestrone Soup with White	Spaghetti Squash with Lentil Marinara	Avocad o Chocol ate Mousse
Day 10			
Mediterra nean Chickpea Salad	Mushroom and Spinach Risotto	Arepas with Spicy Black Beans	Chia Seed Puddin g with Mixed Berries
Day 11			

Chickpeas	Ratatouille	Lentil Shepherd's Pie	Peanut Butter Banana Ice Cream
Day 12			
Banana Walnut Breakfast Cookies	Moroccan Carrot Salad	Coconut Curry Tofu with Vegetables	Coconut Yogurt Parfait
Day 13			
Pineapple Ginger Green Smoothie	Quinoa Tabbouleh Salad	Butternut Squash and Sweet Potato	Oatmeal Energy Balls

Snack Options throughout the weeks:

- Almond Butter Stuffed Dates
- Veggie Sticks with Beet Hummus
- Spiced Pumpkin Seeds
- Sweet Potato and Kale Hash
- Steamed Green Beans with Almond Slivers

This meal plan provides a variety of flavorful and nutritious plant-based meals, ensuring you receive a balanced diet while enjoying delicious and satisfying dishes. Adjustments can be made based on personal preferences and dietary needs

Shopping list Ingredients

Produce:
Bell peppers (assorted colors)
Eggplant
Zucchini
Spinach
Mushrooms (cremini, portobello)
Onions
Garlic
Tomatoes
Carrots
Celery
Kale
Lettuce (romaine, kale)
Avocado
Peach
Apple
Mango
Pineapple

Banana
Berries (strawberries, blueberries, raspberries)
Lemon
Lime
Cilantro
Parsley
Basil

Grains and Legumes:
Quinoa
Lentils
Chickpeas (canned or dried)
Tofu
Brown rice
Whole wheat pasta
Polenta (cornmeal)
Farro
Couscous
Bulgur
Wild rice
Nuts and Seeds:
Walnuts
Almonds
Flaxseeds
Chia seeds
Pumpkin seeds
Dairy and Dairy Alternatives:

Coconut milk (canned)
Almond milk
Coconut yogurt

Pantry Staples:
Olive oil
Balsamic vinegar
Soy sauce (or tamari for gluten-free)
Nutritional yeast
Agave nectar
Tomato paste
Vegetable broth
Canned diced tomatoes
Canned coconut milk
Tahini
Spices and herbs (cumin, paprika, turmeric, chili powder, oregano, thyme, rosemary, etc.)
Salt and pepper
Whole grain flour (for baking)

Other:
Whole grain bread
Pita bread
Tortillas
Arepa flour
Hummus
Olives
Dried fruit (cranberries, raisins)
Dark chocolate (for desserts)
Coconut flakes
Vegetable bouillon cubes

This shopping list covers a wide range of ingredients needed for the recipes in the book, ensuring that you have everything you need to create delicious and nutritious plant-based meals. Adjust quantities based on personal preferences and the number of servings required.

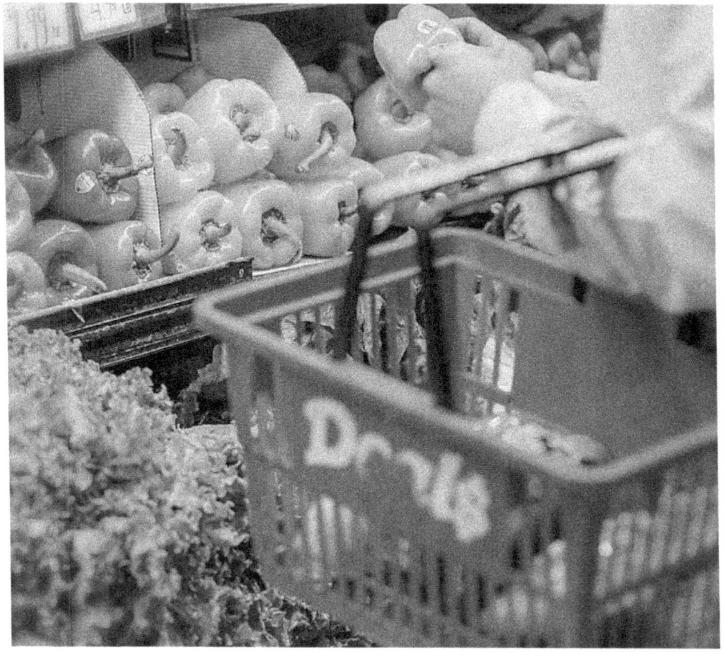

Conclusion

As you reflect on your journey towards embracing a plant-based lifestyle in your later years, take a moment to celebrate your achievements and the positive impact it has had on your health and well-being. You've made significant strides in prioritizing nutritious and wholesome foods that nourish your body and support your vitality.

Through your commitment to plant-based eating, you've not only improved your physical health but also contributed to a more sustainable and environmentally friendly way of living. By choosing plant-based meals, you've reduced your carbon footprint and embraced a lifestyle aligned with your values.

Moreover, your journey has been about more than just food. It's been a journey of self-discovery, empowerment, and growth. You've explored new flavors, discovered exciting recipes, and learned to appreciate the abundance of plant-based ingredients available to you.

As you continue on your plant-based journey, remember to approach it with curiosity, openness, and compassion. Embrace the process of learning and evolving, knowing that every step you take towards a plant-based lifestyle is a step towards greater health, vitality, and well-being.

Celebrate the joy of nourishing your body with plant-based goodness and the sense of connection it brings to your life and the world around you. Your journey is a testament to the power of choice and the transformative impact it can have on your health, happiness, and the planet.

Bonus 1: Nutritional Information For Meals

Quinoa-Stuffed Bell Peppers

Serving Size: 1 serving |Total Calories: 311 kcal
Cholesterol: 0 mg | Fats: Total Fat 3.4 g, Saturated
Fat - not specified
Sodium: 498 mg | Total Carbohydrates: 59 g, | Fiber
11.5 g, Sugar 8.2 g | Protein: 14.4 g

Chickpea and Vegetable Stir-Fry

Serving Size: 1 serving | Total Calories: 315 kcal |
Fats: Total Fat 7.6 g | Saturated Fat 3 g
Sodium: 930 mg | Total Carbohydrates: 50 g, Fiber
12 g, Sugar 9 g | Protein: 20g | Vitamin A 77 IU |
Vitamin C 427 mg | Calcium 21 mg | Iron 30 mg2

Eggplant Parmesan

Serving Size: 1 cup | Total Calories: 317 kcal
Cholesterol: 95 mg | Fats: Total Fat 16.83 g,
Saturated Fat 7.741 g | Sodium: 655 mg
| Total Carbohydrates: 23.15 g | Fiber 2.8 g, Sugar
4.46 g | Protein: 18.88 g | Vitamin D 0 mcg | Calcium
441 mg | Iron 1.91 mg, Potassium 277 mg3

Lentil Shepherd's Pie

Total Calories: 356 kcal | Cholesterol: 0 mg
Fats: Total Fat 7.5 g | Saturated Fats 1.7 g

Sodium: 570 mg |Total Carbohydrates: 48.6 g, Fiber 10.6 g | Protein: 17.1 g | Potassium 1070 mg | Phosphate 300 mg4

Chickpea and Spinach Coconut Curry
Total Calories: 312 kcal | Fats: Total Fat 21 g | Saturated Fat 13 g | Sodium: 817 mg
Total Carbohydrates: 25 g | Fiber 7 g | Sugar 1 g
Protein: 9 g | Vitamin A 130 IU | Vitamin C 8 mg | Calcium 73 mg | Iron 4 mg5

Mediterranean Stuffed Portobello Mushrooms
Serving Size: 1 mushroom (128g) | Calories: 90 kcal|Cholesterol: 0 mg | Fats: Total Fat 2.5g, Saturated Fat 1g | Trans Fat 0g
Sodium: 539mg | Total Carbohydrates: 20g, Fiber 5g | Sugar 5g | Protein: 13g | Vitamin A 9532IU | Vitamin C 25mg | Calcium 231mg | Iron 3mg1

Asian-Inspired Tofu Stir-Fry
Total Calories: 144 kcal | Cholesterol: 0 mg
Fats: Total Fat 6g | Saturated Fat 1g | Trans Fat 0g | Sodium: 557mg | Total Carbohydrates: 15g, Fiber 5g, Sugar 6g | Protein: 9g
Vitamin A 6655IU | Vitamin C 50.2mg, Calcium 42mg | Iron 2.1mg2

Ratatouille
Serving Size: 1 cup (215g) | Total Calories: 140 kcal | Cholesterol: 0 mg | Fats: Total Fat 10g, Trans Fat 0g

Total Carbohydrates: 12g | Fiber 4.1g | Sugar 7.3g |
Protein: 2.4g

Stuffed Acorn Squash with Wild Rice and Cranberries

Total Calories: 388 kcal | Cholesterol: 0 mg
Fats: Total Fat 12g, Saturated Fat 1g, Trans Fat 0g |
Sodium: 10mg | Total Carbohydrates: 69g, Fiber 8g,
Sugar 11g | Protein: 9g | Vitamin A 791IU, Vitamin
C 24mg, Calcium 90mg, Iron 3mg4

Coconut Curry Tofu with Vegetables

Total Calories: 364 kcal | Cholesterol: 0 mg
Fats: Total Fat 22.9g, Saturated Fat Not specified,
Trans Fat 0g | Sodium: 886.4mg
Total Carbohydrates: 26.4g, Sugar 9.2g
Protein: 15.6g
Please note that the information provided is based on
specific recipes and may vary depending on the
exact ingredients and quantities used. For a
complete nutritional profile, it's best to calculate the
values based on the specific recipe you're using. If
you need more detailed information or for other
meals, let me know! Reach out to me at
mariakirby001@gmail.com

14 WEEKS MEAL PLANNER

Days	Breakfast	Lunch	Dinner	Snacks/ Desserts
Mon				
Tues				
Wed				
Thurs				
Fri				
Sat				

Sun				

Days	Breakfast	Lunch	Dinner	Snacks/ Desserts
Mon				
Tues				
Wed				
Thurs				
Fri				
Sat				
Sun				

Days	Breakfast	Lunch	Dinner	Snacks/ Desserts
Mon				
Tues				
Wed				
Thurs				
Fri				
Sat				
Sun				

Days	Breakfast	Lunch	Dinner	Snacks/ Desserts
Mon				
Tues				
Wed				
Thurs				
Fri				
Sat				
Sun				

Days	Breakfast	Lunch	Dinner	Snacks/Desserts
Mon				
Tues				
Wed				
Thurs				
Fri				
Sat				
Sun				

Days	Breakfast	Lunch	Dinner	Snacks/ Desserts
Mon				
Tues				
Wed				
Thurs				
Fri				
Sat				
Sun				

Days	Breakfast	Lunch	Dinner	Snacks/ Desserts
Mon				
Tues				
Wed				
Thurs				
Fri				
Sat				
Sun				

Days	Breakfast	Lunch	Dinner	Snacks/ Desserts
Mon				
Tues				
Wed				
Thurs				
Fri				
Sat				
Sun				

Days	Breakfast	Lunch	Dinner	Snacks/ Desserts
Mon				
Tues				
Wed				
Thurs				
Fri				
Sat				
Sun				

Days	Breakfast	Lunch	Dinner	Snacks/ Desserts
Mon				
Tues				
Wed				
Thurs				
Fri				
Sat				
Sun				

Days	Breakfast	Lunch	Dinner	Snacks/ Desserts
Mon				
Tues				
Wed				
Thurs				
Fri				
Sat				
Sun				

Days	Breakfast	Lunch	Dinner	Snacks/ Desserts
Mon				
Tues				
Wed				
Thurs				
Fri				
Sat				
Sun				

Days	Breakfast	Lunch	Dinner	Snacks/ Desserts
Mon				
Tues				
Wed				
Thurs				
Fri				
Sat				
Sun				

Days	Breakfast	Lunch	Dinner	Snacks/ Desserts
Mon				
Tues				
Wed				
Thurs				
Fri				
Sat				
Sun				

Get the hardcover version for better user experience and more exclusive bonuses including premium color version.